MW00856765

# THE REPRODUCTION OF EVIL:
# A CLINICAL AND CULTURAL PERSPECTIVE

# RELATIONAL PERSPECTIVES BOOK SERIES

STEPHEN A. MITCHELL AND LEWIS ARON
Series Editors

# THE REPRODUCTION OF EVIL
## A CLINICAL AND CULTURAL PERSPECTIVE

### SUE GRAND

**THE ANALYTIC PRESS**

2000    Hillsdale, NJ    London

© 2000 by The Analytic Press, Inc.

All rights reserved. No part of this book may be stored, transmitted, or reproduced in any form whatsoever without the prior written permission of the publisher.

Published by
The Analytic Press, Inc.
   Editorial Offices:
   101 West Street
   Hillsdale, New Jersey 07642
   www.analyticpress.com

   Designed and typeset by Compudesign, Charlottesville, VA.
   Index by Leonard S. Rosenbaum.


**Library of Congress Cataloging-in-Publication Data**

Grand, Sue.
   The reproduction of evil : a clinical and cultural perspective / Sue Grand.
      p.    cm. — (Relational perspectives book series; v. 17)
   Includes bibliographical references and index.
   ISBN 0-88163-261-9
      1. Good and evil—Psychological aspects.   2. Good and evil—Social aspects.   3. Psychoanalysis and culture.   4. Psychic trauma.   I. Title. II. Series.
   BF789.E94 G73 2000
   616.85'8—dc21

                                                                99-462324

Printed in the United States of America

10   9   8   7   6   5   4   3   2   1

In memory of Wendy Greenstone, Bobbye Troutt,
and my grandmother, Jenny:
in death, as in life, they exhort me to pursue justice.

For survivors everywhere,
and for those who do not survive.

Above all,
For Bernie, without whom, not.

# CONTENTS

# ACKNOWLEDGMENTS

GROWING UP IN 1950S SUBURBIA was a study in contradiction. We lived in clean tract houses, on safe and segregated streets. It always seemed like a benign summer, as if there were no human darkness, no zone of human suffering. But if television brought us game shows, it also brought us the unexpurgated newsreels of the Nazi death camps. And as the child of a Jewish father who had participated in the liberation of such camps as an American soldier, the newsreels consolidated what I already knew. The earliest lexicon of my childhood was ordered by my father's memories of Dachau and by his lived amnesias. Through her Holocaust studies, my mother taught me the imperative of remembering history. I was both silenced and challenged by the contradictory edict of my childhood: that I must remember and protest oppression and injustice; that I must live, know nothing, forget.

I was a teenager in the 1960s. Television was *Father Knows Best* and advertisements for household cleansers and appliances. But it was also news footage of Vietnam, civil rights marches, and Mississippi burning. The cultural fabric of forgetting was unravelling in mass protest. It had become possible to think. And then, I learned that an intimate childhood friend was dead of suicide. Sexually abused by her own father, raped by a group of local athletes, silenced in a community of decent neighbors, she took her own life. Her father, an alcoholic, was a combat survivor of World War II: in his "cups" he had always raved about history. Drunk, he would impale his daughter on his own fractured memory of war. Knowing my friend as well as her perpetrator, I reencountered the imagery of my childhood. Now, I began a lifelong inquiry into the survival of malignant trauma, and into the cultural/psychological forces that challenge us to know and to act, even as they exhort us to forget. Over the years, many people have enriched my understanding, laughed with me and cried with me, and have ameliorated my solitude. They are: Judy Alpert, Lurline Aslanian, Patricia Burns, Noa Daskal, Yehuda Daskal, Eve Ensler, Wendy Greenstone, Helga Grunberg, Steve Herman, Howard Jurist, Jennifer Leighton, Peggy Levison, Marylou Lionells, Paul McGowan, Bernie Rous, Jeanne Safer, Jared See, Bonnie See, Lester Shapiro, Joyce Slochower, Barbara Suter, Vivian Rous, Bobbye Troutt, and Ellen Wachtel.

I began treating patients in the late 1970s. At that time, no one mentioned trauma as a causal agent in emotional suffering. By the mid-1980s, a few books had been published, and a few patients began to speak of their history of rape, incest, childhood beatings. These voices resonated with the legacies of my childhood, and they arrested my professional consciousness. To all my patients who struggle with malignant trauma, I am grateful for everything you have taught me, morally as well as clinically. Your courage to speak has induced me to speak on your behalf. And to those patients who have given me permission to tell their stories in this book, thank you. And I am grateful to my analytic supervisors who taught me to empathize and to listen: Mannie Ghent, Bernie Friedland, and Ruth Lesser. I am also grateful to my analytic colleagues whose writings have filled the gap in the analytic literature on trauma: Judy Alpert, Jodie Davies, Mary Gail Frawley, Richard Gartner, Elizabeth Hegeman, Adrienne Harris, Helene Kafka, Helene Nemiroff, Michele Price, Bruce Reis, Sue Shapiro, and many others.

Several years after the completion of my analytic training, Judy Alpert invited me to participate in a trauma study group. A passionate, impeccably ethical activist in trauma studies, Judy was the first to comment on, stimulate, facilitate, and publish my work. She has offered me unfailing support, guidance, and encouragement, and enabled me to consider writing a book. In addition, the other members of my trauma study group, Uli Baer, Claire Cosentino, Michele Price, and Bruce Reis, have stimulated my ideas. When I embarked on my study of evil, Bruce Reis was particularly helpful in locating relevant readings. During this period, Neil Altman and Muriel Dimen were generous and helpful in facilitating and critiquing my writing on trauma.

All of these people inspired me to write about trauma survival. But it was through my singular, ongoing dialogue with Marylou Lionells that I came to write about the perpetration of evil. Over several years, we had dynamic exchanges about the nature of analysis, and whether (and how) psychoanalysis could treat malevolent patients, and the problems of evil. If so, how; if not, why not? In reviewing these dilemmas, I discovered our shared, implicit conviction: that mental health is not simply the capacity to love and to work. It is the struggle to behave with ethical strength on behalf of the other, and for oneself. Repudiating moralism, but unabashedly embracing morality, Marylou freed me to articulate my own clinical and moral perspective on these issues. In addition, she generously read and critiqued numerous versions of this book.

I want to express tremendous gratitude toward my editor, Lew Aron. With his unrestrained enthusiasm, his empathic and incisive critiques, his encyclopedic knowledge of the literature, and his continual encouragement, Lew facilitated my voice and challenged me to write my best book. Working with him was an honor and a delight. I would like also to thank Dorothy Blanchard for her enthusiastic resourcefulness in locating relevant literature, and Jared See for his genial obsessionalism in creating order out of the chaos of my references. And I would like to thank Nancy Liguori at The Analytic Press for her patience, good humor, and excellence in editing. I appreciate Paul Stepansky, Managing Director of The Analytic Press, for valuing the potential of this book.

Finally, I thank my husband, Bernie Rous, optimist, deep thinker, and deep listener, whose patience and kindness make all things possible.

# PREFACE

ALICE'S BODY STANK, AND WITH THIS STENCH SHE INFECTED ME. She lay on the couch, and its fabric absorbed her sweat. Reclusive and obese, she spoke of little else but of food, of body holes, of consuming and excreting, of her mother's hostility and neglect, of an empty purse, of always being "dead broke." It was winter, but when she was present I felt stifled in her sweat. Each session she wore the same polyester clothes; each session they appeared ever more soiled. It was as if she ate, slept, urinated, and defecated in the same clothes, day after day, week after week. I hated her body, and I tried not to smell her. When she left, she was still odiferously present. I aired my room. Now her fecal presence was indistinct, and still I sensed it. When my next patient arrived, I felt vaguely humiliated: would she think this odor emanated from my body? Alice's smell separated me from her and bound me to her. It separated me from my next patient, with whom I sank into an avoidant isolation. I tried to forget Alice's body when she was present. And when I was with my next patient, we would jointly collude in pretending that the smell was not there, because it was somehow unspeakable in its significance. Either it was one of *us*, which was disturbing, or it was my prior patient, which was an intrusion into our private space.

   How could I tell Alice that she stank without evoking a toxic humiliation? How could I continue working with her without telling her? I understood that her body presence was that of a neglected infant. I saw her as unwashed by her mother, left in rank diapers. I imagined that she had been so neglected that she did not know the clean scent of washed bodies and washed clothes. Perhaps as we "worked things through" an organic process of self-care would evolve, and I would no longer struggle with such loathing and disgust.

But the smell overcame me. I felt the need to protect myself and my subsequent patient from Alice's intrusions. Gently, I inquired about her bathing, about her deodorant, and her washing of her clothes, suggesting she did not smell as she might. And I discovered this: that she was not humiliated but gleeful. Yes, she always knew she was rank, she parted crowds, emptied subway seats around her. She loved the power of offending and of paralyzing those whom she offended; she knew that no one who was "civilized" dared to mention her odor. Their silence was her power; their disgust was her vengeance. The human world had rejected and isolated her; she had envied all the attachments from which she was excluded. If they would not love her, she would nonetheless impress herself on them. Indeed, she willfully avoided showering. Sniffing her armpits before leaving her apartment, measuring her own foul ripeness, she pleasurably anticipated the offense she might give throughout the day.

This knowledge cast my neglected patient in a new light. It induced an inquiry into other transgressions, and I discovered that she was a particularly malignant and cunning thief. Alice worked at a poorly paid job, doing home care for the aged. She would visit impoverished, isolated old women and help them cash their social security checks, run their errands, and shop with them. She was chatty and "helpful" and these women loved her. They did not seem alienated by her odor; perhaps they too had longed ceased to bathe. Inevitably, these old women became concerned: they thought their checks were for more money, but the money always seemed to be running short. Already confusional, often in various stages of dementia, they were readily derailed from their own convictions. They would arrive home with a certain amount of money and then be unable to find a portion of it. Alice would patiently help them search their purses. She would "look" under the beds, in the streets in front of the houses. Or she would explain that they were mistaken: the check was really for a smaller amount than they had imagined. Or she told them they had already spent it. The women would become increasingly flustered and upset, anticipating further impoverishment and cognitive disintegration. Bereft and forgotten, these women became ever more dependent. It was Alice who was their comfort, who reassured them, calmed them, and helped them "manage." Each week they were more desperate for her arrival. Losing all doubts in the maze of their own disorientation, they had nothing but faith in Alice. Sometimes they offered her small, poignant gifts for "caring" for them. Slowly, these women ate more and more dog food while Alice grew fatter on the money she had stolen from them after cashing their checks.

She had been stealing this way for at least a year when I confronted her odor. It was this confrontation that precipitated her confession. I had been repelled by her body; I was more repelled by her cruelty and entitlement. I did not attempt to hide my reaction, and insisted that our therapeutic agenda include an end to the thefts and a gradual replacement of these funds. It emerged that she did feel slightly guilty and ashamed. But wasn't she underpaid, exploited by the city for which she worked, starving from maternal neglect? What was their life on dog food compared with her own life? At least *they* had once had a life. If she stole from them, at least she comforted them, returning reliably each week to take care of them. Indeed, she seemed truly fond of her old ladies, and had formed her only relationships with the victims of her theft.

I inquired into her sense of entitlement, and so, the details of the maternal "neglect" emerged. Alice had been beaten and locked in dark closets, emerging from these closets to be shunned by her mother's cold and stony silence. She preferred the beatings to the silence, for the beatings were some form of human interaction. What she feared most was the darkness in the closet, the sound of the door locking, the retreating footsteps, the silence beyond the door as the mother left the house, the fear of the mother returning, the fear that she would never return. Her only companion in the closet was her own urine and feces and sweat: in their odor, she knew she was still living. Once, the mother had left for two days, and Alice was discovered by concerned neighbors. But the neighbors had no recourse: there were no laws then about child abuse, there was no social or familial intervention. And the mother was canny: she threatened Alice if she did not keep silent; she explained Alice's "absences" as "visits to relatives." Worried but impotent, neighbors were doubtless relieved at the "cessation" of abuse.

Then Alice told me this: every week she had been stealing change from the pockets of my coat as it hung in the waiting room. With my change she bought candy, which she hid in her basement room. She had been waiting for me to discover the thefts but I did not, because it is my habit to drop loose change into my pockets, and to remove it when I notice that my pockets are getting full with a certain excessive weight. I do not count the money going in and coming out of my pockets. All of my pockets are in various stages of emptying and filling, and my mind is in a permanent state of vagueness regarding the amount and locus of my funds. Still, I have a satisfying sense of plentitude and resource: something is always full when something else is empty. In searching for something to steal, Alice had encountered the theater of my pockets. She emptied them and they mysteriously refilled. She violated me and took my plenitude with her. And still, the pockets refilled.

My pockets afforded Alice a sense of magical gratification. But there was also the problem of my silence. How was it that I displayed no suspicion, no accusation of theft? She became certain I knew, and, fearful of retribution, she confessed. Had she not been so immersed in her fear of my abandoning her, she would have seen that I had not known, that I would never know. She could have stolen from me forever; it required no stealth. For me to know would have required that I enter some dark internal space of depletion. I refused to let her theft induct me into this space. And so, when she confessed, I was only mildly offended. I had so much, after all, and she had taken so little. I didn't even ask her to repay what she had taken. Increasingly disturbed by my disconnection, she had imagined that I knew, that I laid traps for her, that the most byzantine of punishments awaited her. How absurd it all was: her fear of punishment, her need to be punished; my refusal to punish because the urge toward punishment must arise out of my own depletion.

How had she found us: the old women who *could not know* of her thefts; the therapist *who would not know* of her thefts. There was something about all this knowing and not knowing that was pivotal to her transgressions. I thought again about the way she had pressed her stench into me. When I was silent, she feared that she did not smell, and when she did not smell, she knew *she* was dead. When I was silent, and she knew she smelled, she feared *I* was dead. For weeks, she had escalated the level of her filth. And then there were the thefts in the waiting room, thefts to which I was insensate. She had stolen from me. She had found me oblivious and herself still alive: and so, *I must be dead*. When the pockets refilled, she knew that I was not dead, but alive with cruelty and with vengeance. Which body was living, and which was to be slaughtered?

It was true that she stole a link to my nurturance. It was true that she wanted a relationship grounded in accountability, and that she feared that accountability would result in annihilation. All of this was signified by the stench, by the cash she stole, and the relationships in which she stole it. But there was also something about not-knowing, about the relation between the living and the dead. She not only stole food, she stole *evidence*: what she took were clues to the confusional transactions that suffuse all human cruelty. She took these clues and she left these clues, until I began to think about evil and the problem of human loneliness.

# CHAPTER 1

# AN INTRODUCTION TO MALIGNANT DISSOCIATIVE CONTAGION

LURED BY THE HEROIC AND DEHUMANIZED BY BOOT CAMP, a young man becomes a soldier. If he is a foot soldier, he enters combat, and visions of the heroic recede. Now he is nothing but a student of violence: what he learns are the ways a body can be slaughtered. Severed from everything but command and survival, captive in a universe where murder is sanctioned, and tenderness is not, he evacuates his mind of all human thought. He must move forward into battle, and he does move forward, until that movement itself becomes a hypnotic:

> They marched for the sake of the march. They plodded along slowly, dumbly, leaning forward against the heat . . . just humping, one step and then the next and then another, but no volition, no will, because it was automatic, it was anatomy, and the war was entirely a matter of posture and carriage, the hump was everything, a kind of inertia, a kind of emptiness, a dullness of desire and intellect and conscience and hope and human sensibility [O'Brian, 1990, p. 15].

In the hypnotic numbness of the "hump," there is only war's simple reduction: move forward, kill or be killed. If the soldier lives, he kills. If he dies, he is dead among thousands. And so he kills, mechanically, without hate or desire. He kills, and he knows he kills, but it is a dull and distant knowledge. And then, there is a day when his buddy has died. Now the ubiquity of corpses gives way to a particular dead. Lonely, impotent, excluded from mourning by military stoicism, now, on this day, blood lust may overtake him (Shatan, 1977, 1982, 1986; Nachmani, 1997). The mechanical "hump" becomes a sadistic atrocity. In that atrocity, humanity splits: there are the innocent, there are those who annihilate the innocent; there are those who protect them, and those who fail to protect them.

> Q: What happened then?
> A: Lieutenant Cally walked over to Sergeant Mitchell. They walked backward and started shoving the people into the ditch with their rifles.
> Q: What did you do?
> A. Nothing. I looked away [Hammer, 1971, p. 132].

Men, women, children: in their blood the soldier finds ecstatic self-restitution; in their bodies he evokes every dimension of human suffering. He is exhilarated in brutality, and bankrupt in his judgment. Afterwards, he remembers, and he does not remember. There was no atrocity, but an act of war: the necessary extermination of a network of spies, of armed children, of wombs pregnant, not with fetuses, but with bombs: "I didn't discriminate between individuals in the village, sir. They were all the enemy, they were all to be destroyed, sir" [Lt. William Calley, in Hammer, 1971, p. 263].

As Simenauer (1982) says of Nazi Germany, "No one did any evil; everyone merely performed the highest duty, blindly to obey" (p. 169). And so the soldier commits atrocity, and makes no judgment, or judges it defensible (Stern, 1995). Or he is the bystander, inert, scarred by atrocity's imprint, perhaps judging his paralysis as defensible, or perhaps, as reprehensible. And what of the surviving victim: how does atrocity transmogrify his interior? Will his lived memory become a force of justice, a renewal of violence, or a habitual pattern of revictimization? Or will the survivor become

another bystander, sealed in some paralyzing membrane that pro-
hibits all agency in subsequent encounters with violence? Will he
find that fear

> puzzles the will,
> And makes us rather bear those ills we have
> Than fly to others that we know not of?
> Thus conscience does make cowards of us all,
> And thus the native hue of resolution
> Is sicklied o'er with the pale cast of thought,
> And enterprises of great pitch and moment
> With this regard their currents turn awry
> And lose the name of action
> [*Hamlet,* act 3, scene 1].

This book meditates on these questions; it inquires into the
memory of annihilation, and asks how that memory is lived,
shared, and silenced in the relational nexus of evil. In particular, I
am preoccupied with the way annihilation's memory is transmuted
into the perpetration of evil. I do not presume that all evil is
rooted in a history of trauma survival. Most trauma survivors do
not become perpetrators. But most perpetrators have a history of
malignant trauma, that is, an experience of psychic or physical torture, or both, inflicted by another. I propose that this traumatic history finds a singular articulation in the interpersonal and
intrapsychic operations of evil. This chapter provides a conceptual
introduction to the link between trauma and evil, whereas suc-
ceeding chapters utilize clinical, literary, and cultural material to
elucidate these concepts.

## CATASTROPHIC LONELINESS AND THE
## REPRODUCTION OF EVIL

And so I begin with a look at trauma's core. As Krystal (1988),
Langer (1991, 1995), Felman (1992), Laub (1992), Caruth (1995),
and others suggest, the survival of massive trauma seems to be

characterized by a region of unknowable and unshareable experience. Simply put, there can never be another who can know the survivor in the moment of the "execution itself." In her core, the trauma survivor remains solitary in the moment of her own extinction. No one knew her in the moment when she died without dying; no one knows her now, in her lived memory of annihilation. This place where she cannot be known is one of catastrophic loneliness; it is a solitude imbued with hate and fear and shame and despair. And it is an area of deadness strangely infused with a yearning for life. For unlike the dead, she is at once dead and yet *left alive in the wake of her own destruction*. Death has possessed her in its impenetrable solitude. But life makes her desire to be known in that solitude. When cruelty has collapsed the survivor's pretraumatic self, rebirth is sought in the empathic witnessing of the traumatized self (Langer, 1991, 1995; Caruth, 1995; Laub and Podell, 1995). Because that traumatized self is defined by solitude, the survivor's resurrection requires that she be *known by another in this solitude*, for, as Benjamin (1995) notes, "The sea of death can be crossed only by reaching the other" (p. 186).

But any attempt to know the survivor in the execution itself is to "listen to an impossibility" (Caruth, 1995). How can the survivor be known by another in a moment defined by its loneliness? Who will be the knower and who (and what) will be the known? Loneliness is a space that precludes the presence of another. And this loneliness of the survivor is no ordinary loneliness: it is not merely the "unthought known" (Bollas, 1995) or the "unformulated" in Stern's (1997) sense. This loneliness is not something wordless that can be ultimately rendered in speech. It is *unformulatable: it cannot be represented mutually in linguistic narrative*. Whatever can be known mutually and linguistically about traumatic experience is not death's solitude but something else, some other pain that exists at the perimeter of death. This is annihilation's paradox: that the need to be known continually meets the impossibility of being known. And the need to be known meets, as well, an inner *refusal* to be known. Much as another's empathic understanding is critical for the survivor's resurrection, so that very understanding threatens to renew the survivor's annihilation. Any presumption of knowledge will eviscerate the truth of her loneliness, collapsing the core of her traumatic identity. Loneliness is the sacred container of the survivor's residual sanity; it *is* the survivor's ultimate testimony. It must not and cannot be foreclosed.

Annihilation awakens contradictory desires that can be neither achieved nor surrendered. The survivor's predicament resonates with the schizoid dilemma described by Laing (1960) and Guntrip (1969). What Ulman and Brothers (1988) call the "shattered self" of trauma is suffused with death anxiety, with the sense that there is no self. Such a personality becomes preoccupied with the protection and concealment of the no-self and its deadness, because, paradoxically, deadness and vacuity are the defining qualities of the person's tenuous identity. Other people become figures of hope and dread. While they potentially offer much needed confirmatory evidence of the existence of the self, they nonetheless threaten to eclipse the no-self with the larger presence of their own identities. Without confirmatory contact with another, the no-self will wither and die; with it, it will be annihilated. In the presence of such acute existential anxieties, there is a "pre-experiential motivational push, a drive, for a meeting of minds," which "meets a drive to remain hidden, an isolate, unfound and untouched by others" (Aron, 1996, p. 80). In Pizer's (1999) sense, this is an area of the self that seeks and resists therapeutic "negotiation." The difficulty that the schizoid process poses for analyst and patient (see Guntrip, 1969, on the schizoid compromise) increases when this process originates in malignant trauma: the remoteness of the no-self is excacerbated, as is the impossibility of being known. And yet, the desire to be known is imbued with that urgency which attends the final moments before slaughter.

How does humanity metabolize this dilemma? What I propose throughout these essays is this: that evil is an attempt to answer the riddle of catastrophic loneliness. Unlike all other forms of human interaction, evil alone bears witness to the contradictory claims of solitude and mutuality that haunt traumatic memory. The reproduction of evil is the survivor's continual reentry into the moment of execution, where "death is the irreducible common denominator of men" (King, 1963, p. 117). The survivor has been waiting to be known, not merely in the *memory* of the execution, but in the execution *itself*. It is here that her solitude was defined; it is here that she attempts to be known in her solitude. For torture is a transaction between what Sullivan (1953) calls the "not me" and the "not" other. And it is also an "I–it" relation (Buber, 1923, 1947) in which the ego uses another as a thing. Only in the context of evil is it possible to achieve radical contact with another *at the pinnacle of loneliness and at the precipice of death*. Only perpetrator and bystander recreate and encounter the no-self of torture's vacuity, and only they can be *in the presence of that no-self without any pretense of knowing it. In perpetrator and bystander, there is neither the desire for, nor the illusion of "understanding" the no-self. In the perpetrator-bystander-victim relation, the no-self is in the presence of others who confirm the truth of catastrophic loneliness, even as these others do not know this loneliness.*

Through revictimization, through a renewed link to a perpetrator, some survivors attempt to be seen in the area of the no-self. Through perpetration, the survivor who becomes a perpetrator attempts to share his no-self by evacuating it into his victim. In both revictimization and perpetration, *there is a meeting which is no meeting in the execution itself*. This is mankind's nearest approximation of the mutual recognition of solitude: the mutual encounter of torture inevitably collapses into torture's mutual isolation. In a sense, a shared encounter with the no-self can only be found in the treacherous and elliptical loop of destruction. From this perspective we can understand the psychoanalytic dynamism that Benjamin (1999) describes:

> [T]he point at which the patient presents the real difficulty that needs mending, really is often experienced as the moment of maximum attack on our subjectivity (as analysts and as persons). This destruction is inevitable when we work in "basic fault" areas, where traumatic repetition is so emotionally powerful that understanding appears to the patient as useless [p. 203].

Thus, in a myriad of ways, victims return to their tormentors "because being misrecognized feels so much more secure than being unrecognized and unknown" (Nachmani, 1995, p. 430). In this return to the tormentor, the survivor–perpetrator imagines the I–it relation of cruelty fantastically transformed into a paradoxical form of confirmatory relatedness.

In comparison to torture's intrigues, benign relationships can only approximate a memory of the execution, not the execution itself. As Benjamin (1999) notes, "When we work on this fault line, simple recognition is no longer possible, and the effort to remain good, caring, and empathic will only exacerbate the dilemma" (p. 203). In empathic contexts, the survivor will attempt to convey her own traumatic experience, and the other will attempt to understand and heal this experience. Human comfort and human communion will have considerable healing effects. But benign relations cannot transact the region of catastrophic loneliness. Measuring "life in coffee spoons" (Eliot, 1922), measuring death with mere compassion, presuming to know that solitude which cannot be known, they eviscerate the truth of that loneliness.

But evil seduces with its perverse promise of recognition. Evil will always be constituted so that victim after victim is accompanied by her perpetrator to the obscure solitude of extinction. In each new victim, the perpetrator shares his own catastrophic loneliness, in what Bollas (1995) calls the "companionship of the dead." Evil always reaches its terminus in shared loneliness and in the shared disappearance of selves.[1]

Thus, there is a thin edge that forms between the intensely shared experience of torture and the utter bankruptcy of its isolation. If torture precipitates what Fromm-Reichman (1959) called "uncanny loneliness," then the repetition of torture signifies both a shared flight from, and a shared renewal of, that loneliness. In a masterful compromise formation, the survivor-cum-perpetrator

---

1. For, as Bion (1965) and Grotstein (1990) have suggested, destruction is a force of nothingness that subjects human experience to a centripetal pull into the void. Man's elemental hate, envy, and greed (Freud, 1930; Klein, 1935, 1940, 1955) are embedded in this force of nothingness. But, as Greenberg and Mitchell (1983) note, the nothingness of destruction is not an instinct. It is a perverse hungering for an object, as a reprieve from the objectlessness of annihilation (Fairbairn, 1952a, b; Guntrip, 1971).

devises interpersonal dynamisms that are a shared enactment of her impossible desires.[2] These enactments of solitude must involve horrific and compelling encounters and elisions in human dialogue. Through the victim's mind and body, the survivor–perpetrator registers his longing for the absent other, "who could have and should have been there" (Benjamin 1995, p. 193) in the moment of execution. Through the disappearance of the victim's interior, the perpetrator recreates the missing other who is *never* there and can *never* be there. The survivor works out his trauma on the human race by "trying to bring others to an equivalent Fall" (Bollas, 1995, p. 1184): he lives, masters, transforms, and reobliterates the forgotten forms of his own traumatic past. And the no-self of survival is sustained by the imminence of contact, while evading the dangerous properties of contact by extinguishing the other before too much contact is made (see Laing [1960], Winnicott [1960], and Guntrip [1969]).

In the treatment of evil, the therapist must not imagine that a human, narrative relationship with the patient can fully cure what evil cannot solve: the solitary dread of annihilation. For the survivor of malignant trauma, despair looks backwards toward loss and vanished memory, and dread is "an apprehension of the future, a presentiment of a something which is nothing" (Kierkegaard, 1937, p. 38). The survivor exists between the memory of one death and the anticipation of another. He is caught in that force that

> has already devoured the person or the realness of the person. Now it devours the unperson or unrealness of the nonperson. It devours the shell that is left, the counterpart of the person, the empty phony version; the dead false self [Eigen, 1996, p. 106],

and so, that grief which the survivor must hold is no ordinary grief. She may repeatedly seek the bad faith of forgetfulness, in

---

2. These dynamisms are presymbolic forms (see Segal, 1957) of enactments (on enactments, see Bromberg, 1998; Chused, 1991; Davies and Frawley, 1994; Hirsch, 1993; Jacobs 1986; Loewenstein, 1956; MacLaughlin, 1991, Renik, 1993).

which one denies death and becomes both the deceiver and the deceived (Sartre, 1981). The survivor is torn between those conditions that Heidegger (1962) called mindfulness and forgetfulness. In the solitary condition of mindfulness, one confronts and lives with dread and the memory of nothingness. One seeks an authentic present poised between the memory and the anticipation of death. Mindfulness is a condition of agonized wakefulness, in which the survivor mourns "a loss that cannot be undone with retribution or even justice" (Harris, 1997, p. 35). In that mourning, there will always be an element of despair. But despair is that emotion which "forces one to come to terms with one's destiny. . . . It is the great enemy of pretense. . . . Despair is not freedom itself, but is a necessary preparation for freedom" (May, 1981, p. 235). And so, the perpetrator's redemption can only be located in a condition of mindfulness. Partly healed through human communion, aspects of her loneliness will remain incurable. In an effective treatment, loneliness will always continue to defy meaning-making, but will not be malevolent in its aspect.

If we view evil as an attempt to register something solitary and unknowable in the human condition, then we begin to grasp why a sense of mystery pervades any encounter with it. And we do not risk committing what Lanzmann (1995) calls the "obscenity of understanding": the tendency to eviscerate evil by theorizing its interior. Rather, we know that as we draw closer to malevolence, its secrets will elude us. We can investigate evil and retain evil's raw edge: that which cannot be known, articulated, or forgiven.

## MALEVOLENCE AND THE DISAVOWAL OF MALEVOLENCE

It is the Devil's cleverest guile to convince us that he does not exist [Baudelaire].

Generation after generation, mankind has turned against itself in cruelty: in the familial violations of rape, child abuse, child neglect, and spouse battering; in the anonymity of violent crime;

in the mass depredations of war, genocide, racism. Generation after generation, evil has assumed subtle, pedestrian forms. Sometimes sadistic, but more often banal, these interpersonal acts may be perpetrated with *or* without the conscious intent to destroy. Evil seems to be everywhere. And even as it is everywhere, it is everywhere denied: perpetrator and bystander collude in its obfuscation. Indeed, mankind seems to

> have mouths, but cannot speak,
> eyes but cannot see;
> They have ears, but cannot hear,
> . . . . . . . . . . . . .
> They can make no sound in their throats
> [Psalm 115, verses 5–7].

Silence is the facilitator of destruction; it is through denial that evil consolidates its power. Evil tends to be brazen in its presence and yet radical in its concealment, so that, "Once more the storm is howling and half hid" (Yeats, 1933, p. 185). As Arendt argued in 1955 and 1963, evil degrades all truth to meaningless trivialities; it utilizes "language rules" and "holes of oblivion" to marshall its force in a culture of lies: "War is Peace. Freedom is Slavery. Ignorance is Strength" (Orwell, 1949, p. 7).

The diabolic is an arena of disorientation and confusion in which truth is lost, becoming unrecognizable even when seen (see Grotstein, 1979; Bollas, 1992, 1995). This arena is the perpetrator's cloak of invisibility, the evacuation of the victim's mind, the bystander's refusal to acknowledge sin (Coser, 1969; Peck, 1983). Throughout human history, the truth of evil is occluded; the tyrant finds his permit in mankind's credulity: "I shall present propagandistic grounds for starting the war (with Poland); whether they are believable is irrelevant. The victor will not be asked later whether or not he told the truth" (Hitler, 1939, as quoted in Gebhardt, 1970).

This passivity creates a culture of silence. In this culture of silence, the victim of malignant trauma is subject to double shock: the violation of body/psyche and the violation of memory (see Alpert, 1994; also Frankel's [1998] discussion of Ferenczi). She enters a state of affective flooding, catalyptic passivity, and cognitive and motoric paralysis (Krystal, 1976, 1988; Herman, 1992; Van der Kolk, 1996). Before the perpetrator's (and bystander's) denials, she finds her reality bewildered, and is often impotent in her confusion (Ferenczi, 1932; Kramer, 1983; Hegemon, 1995; Kafka, 1995; Grand, 1995, 1997a, b; Shapiro, 1997; Slavin, 1997; Gartner, 1999; etc.). Thus the politics of evil extinguishes her agency, reducing her to simple prey (see also Goldberg, 1996).

In this theater of illusion, the victim is lost. And in this theater of illusion, the victim is defined. How then shall she seek justice? Justice requires knowledge, and knowledge is undone in a culture of lies. Confounded by evil's brilliant obscurantism, justice founders, slow-moving, belated, its language insufficient to its adversary: "The trick . . . was to ignore any facts—whether they pertained to atrocities, rumors of concentration camps, or starvation—that would complicate the [U.S.] policy goal of not getting involved. . . . I got fed up. . . . Every day, it was lies" (Kenny, on Bosnia, in Maas, 1996, pp. 62–63).

In this obfuscation of the truth, evil eludes accountability and justice. Secrecy, concealment, denial, ambiguity, confusion: these are Satan's fellow travelers, requiring elaborate interpersonal and intrapsychic collusion between perpetrators and bystanders. The operations of silence potentiate evil and remove all impediments from its path.

While much has been written about the patterns of interpersonal collusion that faciliate evil and obstruct justice (see Lifton, 1986; Staub, 1989; Herman, 1992; Goldberg, 1996; Baumeister, 1997; etc.), a gap remains in the psychodynamic conceptualization of this collusion. With the exception of Bollas's (1995) work, not-knowing and not-seeing are generally regarded as a strategic surface for evil's more complex depths. Not-knowing tends to be regarded as a separate, simpler variable intersecting with man's dark internal forces. Thus, for example, the Serbian eradication of the mass graves of genocide is perceived as a strategic evasion of accountability. Or the apparent ignorance of "good Germans" during the Nazi regime is attributed to a desire for security in the prewar and war years (for an exception, see Goldhagen, 1996).

Herman (1992) argues that "in order to escape accountability for his crimes, the perpetrator does everything in his power to promote forgetting" (p. 8). Such interpretations are essential and accurate, but incomplete. From my perspective, the disavowal of evil and the perpetration of evil are not separate variables representing surface and depth. Rather, they are a singular manifestation of traumatic memory; together they *are* the deep structure of evil. From this vantage point, there is deep significance to Herman's (1992) perception that "the study of psychological trauma has a curious history—one of episodic amnesia.... Though the field has in fact an abundant and rich tradition, it has been periodically forgotten and must be periodically reclaimed" (p. 7).

## Malignance, Disavowal, and Developmental Regression

Earlier, I suggested that the evil act originates in an enactment of the survivor–perpetrator's unknowable core. Here, I argue that the unknowability that compels evil likewise impels the collusive disavowal of that evil. Together with its "uncanny emotions" (Sullivan, 1953) of hate, shame, terror, and despair, catastrophic loneliness defies reflection, word, and narrative. It cannot fully enter recorded human history. If the vortex of solitude is hidden from mutual knowledge by virtue of its very unknowability, then its malign enactment must likewise be in a state of disappearance. Wherever evil occurs, systemic ambiguity, denial, and obscurity will attend it.

This collusive trend toward concealment proceeds not only from evil's intrinsic unknowability, but also from the peculiarities of that developmental regression which follows upon massive trauma. For trauma is met and endured by a psyche that is creative in the exigencies of survival. Under threat of annihilation, the mind mobilizes primitive defenses, perceptions, cognitions, and affects (which originate in normal infancy and early childhood) in an attempt to metabolize that which cannot be borne. As I demonstrate in chapters 4, 5, and 6, these primitive defenses involve an autistic retreat from the human other, and an incapacity to know both history and agency. Within such primitive modalities, execution's moment is transformed in infinite layers of protest, perception, and disappearance. The result is a traumatized area of the self that attests to execution's reality, even as it obscures that reality.

Ordinary human infancy is rooted in the fragility and dependence of the human body. As a result, early psychological development originates in the need for sustenance (physical and emotional) and in the fear of extinction; it is preoccupied with life and death. In these preoccupations, there is an inherent narcissism: the survival of the self occludes all empathic concerns for the human other. With growth, there is an increasing sense of security; annihilation anxieties recede, although they never fully subside; empathic concern for the human other awakens as mortal terror recedes. Enduring massive trauma reacquaints the psyche with the nearness of extinction. Once again, the human mind is preoccupied with the terror of nonbeing. Once again, the mind asks: will the world feed me or starve me, hold me or attack me? But because the no-self of trauma has already met death, these questions have acquired a new increment of dread. They are no longer balanced by the countervailing hope, love, and play of normal infancy, but become something darker. They are asked with despair, with an assurance that goodness has absented itself, with a conviction that the world "out there" is one of danger. Already isolated by catastrophic loneliness, the no-self perceives the human world as one of imminent badness. As Alford (1997, 1998) notes in his neo-Kleinian analysis of evil, the no-self manages its dread of death by mobilizing pathological forms of early developmental modalities. Destructive defenses surface to metabolize dread. In my own language, I would say that the perpetrator's no-self further consolidates its retreat from I–thou relatedness by embracing the insularity of pathological narcissism. And this no-self attempts to escape its own insularity by inscribing its loneliness on the victim.

In my view, this retreat does not simply potentiate destructive defense mechanisms. This retreat is an entry into early developmental modalities that *lack the capacity for historicity and personal accountability*. In pathological regression, life is lived in an immediate present. There is no experienced "I" who can reflect on, and remember, her own history; there is no past or future to be reflected on or anticipated. And there is no "I" who initiates life events, hence, there is no sense of personal, moral accountability for one's acts. Instead of history, there is a "continual defensive recasting of the past" (Ogden, 1989, p. 13), in which "the significance of facts for truth undergoes eclipse or extinction" (Grotstein, 1981, p. 93). As a result, the perpetrator's depravities coalesce in an internal environment in which the act is *not really real, not really evil, or not really mine* (for an in-depth discussion of this phenomenon, see chapter 4). The evil act is therefore internally obscured and *interpersonally obscuring;* the perpetrator's relational field is infected with the disappearance of history. Transacting the world through malignant operations that erase history even as such history is made: this is the perverse result of massive trauma intersecting with destructive psychic forces and with developmental regression (for discussions of the link between the regression, destruction, and the occlusion of history, see chapters 4, 5, and 6).

Because evil is rooted in particular types of developmental regression and because evil is a product of trauma's unknowable core, an evil act defies the type of shared, historical narration that can be mutually reflected on, remembered, spoken of, objectified, and interpreted. The evil act is intrinsically elusive. While its impact on the victim is stunning, permanent, and incontestable, the evil act seems ephemeral and fraught with ambiguity.

### Systemic Collusion: The Appearance and Disappearance of Evil

Within human culture, the *truth of evil seems to be in a continuous state of appearance and disappearance.* The discovery of evil and the disavowal of that evil is an ongoing process that obtains wherever evil is perpetrated. While this process is transacted on the victim's mind and body, it is potentiated, refracted, and sustained in the family and culture. Systemically, the facts of evil seem to press toward communal knowledge, just as some counterforce undermines the emergence of such knowledge. Emergent knowledge seems like a shape shifter: sometimes located in the perpetrator, but more often in the victim, it resides, as well, in the just bystander. Thus, perpetrators are often flagrantly public in their acts; clues are blatant, as if perpetrators want to be caught. And yet these clues are often met by such stunning denials, that we must question the culture's willful evasion of knowledge. At other times, the victim cries out to be heard, even as the perpetrator eradicates all evidence of the crime. Kosovo refugees emerge with stories of genocide, even as the evidence of this genocide is lost in the eradication of mass graves. Incest survivors attest to their victimization, but incest is committed in the night and obscured by the family's nocturnal sleep; no one knows, and the perpetrator seems quite normal in the morning. Thus the familial and cultural memory for evil seems to be a systemic process in which awakening alternates with obfuscation. Facts about evil emerge, and call for action. And the facts recede into the unknown, intervention falters, and the prevailing myth is that *nothing is really happening.*

This systemic enactment is a precise reflection of the survivor-perpetrator's internal struggle between the desire to be known, the fear of being known, and the impossibility of being known. And it is a precise mirroring of developmental regression with its attendant loss of history and agency. When the family or culture reflects these dynamisms, when the communal history of evil is one in which truth continually appears and disappears, humanity is testifying to the paradox of the perpetrator's no-self. If trauma survival is a "mutually obscuring relationship between being alive and being dead" (Ogden, 1997, p. 61), in which the survivor "cannot historicize his experience [because he remains] anchored in a moment of cruelty and cannot turn perception into memory" (Auerhahn and Laub, 1987, p. 327), then the cultural context of victimization is a larger refraction of this mutually obscuring relationship. Malevolence is inextricably linked to a relational system in which there is a continuous "retrospective falsification of the past" (Bromberg, 1994, p. 537) and a continuous erasure of the present. Its present is obscured and its past is forgotten: by its nature, evil eclipses the very history it is making. Events are entered into history and simultaneously evacuated from history.

This erasure of history is not simply a strategy for reducing conflict and allowing evil to proceed unimpeded, although it has that function. Rather, it is the *shared cultural experience of trauma's unknowability, as well as a shared attempt at metabolizing and redissociating overwhelming affects of hate, shame, despair, and fear.* (For a discussion of dissociation, see, e.g., Krystal, 1976; Herman, 1992; Davies and Frawley, 1994.) For this shared experience to occur, the perpetrator must solicit victim, bystander, and culture to collude in the disavowal of evil. Inevitably, the perpetrator finds her own denial mirrored, echoed, and calcified in others' disavowal of inhuman events.[3]

Thus the interdependence of malevolence and obscurity is an inevitability wherever evil originates in trauma survival. So ubiquitous is this process that it must be named. I refer to it as *malignant dissociative contagion*; the essays in this volume are devoted to the vicissitudes of this contagion.[4]

Malignant dissociative contagion is more than a collusive obliteration of evil's presence. Although I have emphasized evil's intrinsic tendency toward the erasure of knowledge and history, malignant dissociative contagion is not simply characterized by the forces of numbing, concealment, and denial. Rather, it is a dialectical system. The field of evil is certainly characterized by torpor, numbness, concealment, and destruction of evidence, as well as by isolating and obscuring operations. But this field is also character-

---

3. Others' disavowal is not simply a reflection of the perpetrator's no-self. It stems from the ubiquitous human fear of the no-self, from our dread of death, from our own internal dynamisms of not-knowing. In the case of Alice (see the Preface), my own fear of depletion derives from the dread of nothingness; my obliviousness and disavowal follow from that dread.

4. In its qualities of denial, malignant dissociative contagion bears resemblance to Howell's (1996) concepts of "group compartmentalization" and "collective dissociation" in sadomasochistic transactions. In its nonreflective tendency toward the discharge of raw impulse, this field resonates with Freud's (1921) description of group psychology and primary process and with Hopper's (1995) notion of the incohesion group, in which annihilation and fragmentation are defended against through fusion, loss of boundaries, and resultant chaos and confusion. As Robins and Post (1997) might suggest, this group process is impelled by a quest to make meaning out of the meaningless, through the rationalization of malevolence.

ized by heightened awareness and vigilance, vociferous claims to truth and knowledge, exhortations to communal awakening and action, and by heroic acts in which those who perform them feel acutely awake and alive. While perpetrators tend to persist in mystifications and lies, and victims in pursuit of action and knowledge, clarity may reside in the perpetrator: "That day in My Lai, I was personally responsible for killing about 25 people. Personally. Men, Women. From shooting them, to cutting their throats, scalping them. . . . I did it" (Simpson in Bilton and Sim, 1992, p. 7), even as obscurity resides in the culture that contains the perpetrator.

Knowing and not-knowing shift their form and locus throughout the perpetrator, bystander, victim system. Regardless of where knowing or not-knowing is situated, perpetrator, bystander, and victim influence one another's behavior, perceptions, emotions, and states of consciousness. As a labyrinth of intrapsychic operations and interpersonal transactions, malignant dissociative contagion is a system of "mutual influence" (Beebe and Lachmann, 1988; Aron, 1996; Bromberg, 1998). In mutual influence systems, persons unconsciously act upon one another. Here, there is frequently an asymmetry in power (Aron, 1996); someone in a position of dominance inevitably fails to achieve *empathic recognition for the other's autonomous human existence or feeling states.* As Aron (1996) suggests, perpetual systems of mutual influence are systems of inherent danger: "If two people do not acknowledge each other as separate autonomous subjects, then in one way or another they are dominating or submitting to each other" (pp. 150–151). Or, as Bach (1994) puts it, "the unilaterally imposed fantasy is the hallmark of an act of violence."

## DEFINING HISTORY IN THE CONTEXT OF HUMAN MALEVOLENCE

In proposing a theory of evil predicated on the eradication of history, one must ask, what is history? In my view, the understanding and treatment of evil must be rooted in a view of history that is neither positivist nor constructivist. Neither term is adequate to the paradoxical nature of traumatic experience: that it is absolute and immutable, interpretable and unknowable. Indeed the treatment of trauma and evil challenges us to formulate a new epistemological paradigm for psychoanalysis (see chapter 3).

In my view, to know history is to recognize that events are locatable in time, causally related, really real, predicated on agency, and exist both inside and outside of the self. Phenomenologically, events are located in the present or past, and are understood as impacting the future. Most important, these events are experienced as having a certain "objective" corporeal existence outside of the self, even as the self-other relation filters and interprets events. The sense of time and of objective external existence result in a conviction that events are absolute and unchangeable, and possess some essential independence from the subject who interprets it. The sense of time and space allows events to be associated with agency, and allows truth to bear simultaneous markers of objectivity and subjectivity, to be both metaphoric and literal. The true history of past events is at once hard and soft, inner and outer, known and unknowable. Further, there is an empathic capacity to envision these external events from the subjective perspective of another. This capacity for multiple perspective taking occurs without collapsing either the experience of the self or the experience of the other. And it occurs without collapsing the absolute nature of the events being interpreted.

This capacity for historicity (which evolves from the depressive modality—see chapters 4, 5, and 8) is critical to a fundamentally cohesive self, to the evolution of an experienced "I," to empathic human discourse, and, specifically, to evil's accountability. It stands as a powerful opposing force to that destructive force which "goes on working after it destroys existence, time and space" (Eigen, 1996, p. 35, discussing Bion). If evil consumes all, even consuming itself consuming, then intersubjective history attempts to retrieve truth from the void. And the truth that is retrieved remains a paradoxical truth: it is one which can and *cannot* be known, and which must be held in mourning and despair.

## COLLUSION VERSUS CULPABILITY

In treating malignant dissociative contagion, the analyst not only treats the malevolent character; she treats the relational field in which this character is licensed. In this process, the victim's dissociative collusion must be examined. There are times to investigate the victim's obscurantist approach to knowledge, evidence, and history. We may discover that she is actually occluding *the perpetrator's own moral and agentic knowledge*, and may thereby potentiate the perpetrator's destructiveness. When exploring the victim's role in her own annihilation, it is important to remember the perspectives of Aron (1996) and Goldner (1998) regarding systems of mutual influence. In their view, interpersonal interactions are always bidirectional in their effects, but the person in superior power bears exclusive culpability for destructiveness. The view of Aron and Goldner provides an excellent way to understand malignant dissociative contagion; it allows us to examine the victim's role in this contagion without "blaming the victim." Here, perpetrator, bystander, and victim can be seen as mutually influencing each other's internal states and external behaviors. But *only the perpetrator and bystander are culpable for the act of evil*. The victim commands our compassion. Writing about intimate violence, Goldner (1998) forcefully emphasizes the distinction between psychological interdependence and individual responsibility, arguing that the perpetrator of violence bears sole responsibility for that violence:

> To argue that partners mutually *participate* in an interactional process does not mean they are mutually *responsible* for it, or for its catastrophic outcome. . . . on the question of safety, there must be no compromise or ambiguity . . . [we must have] a zero tolerance for violence [Goldner, 1998, pp. 266–267].

I applaud Goldner's position and share it throughout this book.

## CLINICAL, LITERARY, AND CULTURAL MATERIAL

In each of the forthcoming chapters, conceptual perspectives are extensively illustrated with clinical, literary, and cultural material. Before moving further into clinical material, a word about confidentiality. While the essential truth of clinical data has been kept intact, I have altered, disguised, and confabulated nonessential details to conceal patient identity. With regard to gender, I have been careful to avoid the male perpetrator–female victim split. There are an equal number of female and male perpetrators and male and female victims. Throughout my discussions, I alternate pronouns to further avoid the male–female, abuser–victim split. With regard to race: the perpetrators here are from diverse ethnic backgrounds, but all are white; their victims are ethnically and racially diverse.

# CHAPTER 2

# LONELINESS AND THE ALLURE
# OF BODILY CRUELTY

❧

JAMES WOULD CRY OUT IN HIS SLEEP. Sometimes there was an image: a family eating, a piece of furniture, a playing field, an aisle in a drug store. Innocuous, unworthy of terror, these images accrued horror like a flash fire. Then there were the other times, when a cry welled up in his body, vacant of image or context. For years, he had suffered his night terrors and insisted they meant nothing.

His mother too had awakened in the night. She was an Armenian whose family had been massacred by the Turks years before she came to America, where James was born. This much he knew, although he did not know how he knew it; he knew nothing more and did not wish to hear it. He had reached the age of sixty-five, had cared tenderly for his dying mother, and for his mother's dying sister, and yet he could tell me nothing about their life in Armenia.

He said he came to therapy because he was lonely, although he did not know why: he had a good marriage, children, grandchildren. He was a loyal and gentle man, dispensing small kindnesses, living an unexamined life. It was his wife who had always been concerned about the screaming; it was she who had insisted that he speak of the genocide in treatment. *She* was a "thinker" and a reader of books. *He* just wanted to chat about the ordinariness of living: retirement, marital skirmishes, his children, his ailments.

Perhaps, he conceded, he missed his mother, his aunt, his father, and some of his deceased friends. When he spoke of them, his eyes filled with tears. But the massacre of the Armenians meant nothing; he mentioned it only in deference to his wife. Friendly, good-natured, and perhaps a little sad, he desired a simple escape from his loneliness.

His loneliness was familiar, an old state now becoming an intolerable shadow. Professing to know nothing of the Armenian genocide, his loneliness was a link to the massacre: to the unknown dead, to the absent selves and absent stories hidden inside his mother and his aunt. He had always been a passive, kind man: he had sought to know his mother and his aunt through a lifetime of fearful identifications and compulsions. But when he was younger and his loneliness had become too acute, he had tried to assuage his loneliness through the sexual violation of a woman's body.

In the banality of his analytic conversation, in the pedestrian images of his night terrors, in his sparse stories of Armenia: here there was absence, a gap, a margin empty of meaning. In treatment, the story of genocide would acquire raw detail, it would assume narrational shape and meaning. But for James, an infinitude of facts and stories and words would fail to resurrect the missing aspects of his mother and his aunt. To find his mother and his aunt: this was an imperative. Once he sought them in acts of sexual violation. At treatment's end, he would cling to them through a bodily residuum of remorse and loneliness. Where he had been obsessively sexual, he would become utterly impotent. This sexual dysfunction would represent his penance and their memorial: he would refuse all analytic and medical intervention for it. With memory imprinted on his body, he would be less lonely. And when he was lonely, that loneliness would be full with a rich, human significance.

How did he arrive at this impotence? The road to this symptom began in our analysis of his nightmares and bodily stories, through his banal conversation and his sexualized transference. Through this analysis we met his mother and his aunt in Armenia. We envisioned two girls, one 16, one 14, engaged in the business of living: working, playing, cooking, eating. And then a cataclysmic moment when pure fear infused every aspect of their universe: cruelty was absolute, the world ran with blood. Somehow, years later, they arrived in America. His mother married; her sister did not. Together, they resumed cooking, cleaning, eating, walking, working, as if nothing had happened. They neither remembered nor forgot. At night, daily life was preempted by fear. The aunt was an insomniac; the mother slept but woke up screaming. It was this gap between the ordinariness of living and the imminence of annihilation that James brought to his analysis. Through it, we discovered that reenactments of rape were his testimonial to genocide. As he came to know himself in this bodily evidence, his loneliness deepened in its meaning and assumed the painful aspect of mourning and guilt.

## GENOCIDAL MEMORY, AND THE BODY AS WITNESS

Malignant trauma places its survivor at the precipice of death: not the quiescent death of an integrated surrender, but that "violent, dark revolt of being" (Kristeva, 1980, p. 229) that occurs during psychic or physical torture. At such moments, the victim encounters "nature's dreaded forces" and those "great necessities of fate against which there is no remedy" (Freud, 1927). Here, one does not "merely" encounter death. One encounters the knowledge that others are *absolutely present* in one's torture and *absolutely absent* in human compassion. During the "execution," the "wish for life elicits no response from the executioner" (Laub and Auerhahn, 1993, p. 991): no one recognizes the other; it is a moment without mirror and without exchange. One is never seen or known in the moment of execution. In that refusal of all human recognition,

> Things fall apart; the centre cannot hold
> Mere anarchy is loosed upon the world,
> The blood-dimmed tide is loosed, and everywhere
> The ceremony of innocence is drowned;
> [Yeats, "The Second Coming," 1921].

Where the "centre cannot hold," nothingness and meaning-lessness (Grotstein, 1990) arise. Memory of trauma contains an "empty circle" (Laub and Podell, 1995), a "world of horrific boundlessness" (Eigen, 1996, p. 106). In the aftermath of such dis-integration, there is no knower and there is no known: one's very mind has been evacuated of its own defining moment, the moment of one's death. Victimization is a relation defined by its intersub-jective lapse, by its failure of human intercourse, by the absence of all witness (Scarry, 1985; Laub and Podell, 1995; Walsh, 1996). And it is defined by an absenting of the self, by a dissociation that "involves the foreclosure, not the elaboration of psychic contents" (Davies and Frawley, 1994, p. 66). As Laub and Podell suggest (1995, p. 1002), "There can be no testimony to death": it is located outside of human awareness and dialogue.

Those human atrocities that can be neither seen nor heard in the survivor's testimony actually retain their force through narra-tive absence, for this very silence opens up a terrifying imaginary space in the next generation (Felman, 1992; Caruth, 1995; Langer, 1995). Through this fantasy space, the son of a survivor enters his parents' chasm of infinite grief. He creates events and experiences to fill an existential void (see Gampel, 1982; Kestenberg, 1982); he attempts to place the lonely self of trauma into imaginary relation with another *who was there in the execution itself.* To live in the wake of the survivor's memory is to offer one's own interior as atrocity's imaginative witness and respondent (Bergmann, 1983, 1985; Fresco, 1984). Thus, the parent–child/survivor–witness encounter links a solitary execution to recorded human history, making memory real and known:

> [S]omewhere, far away, another cry mourns toward me, another which is the same, the same cry uttered, sung by another voice. As the reply ends, a certitude . . . comes to me that now it has happened. Nothing more. Just this, and in this way—now it has happened . . . that happen-ing which gave rise to my cry has only now, with the rejoinder, really and undoubtedly happened [Buber, 1923, pp. 1–2].

Through art, through relatively benign symptoms and enactments, subsequent generations offer some of the resonance and reprieve of witnessing.

But still, the parental figure is unfound: she has been consumed and evacuated by the execution itself. To bond with this missing parent is to be linked to nothingness, to fear and desolation:

What are the roots that clutch, what branches grow
Out of this stony rubbish? Son of man,
You cannot say, or guess, for you know only
A heap of broken images, where the sun beats,
And the dead tree gives no shelter, the cricket no relief,
And the dry stone no sound of water.
. . . . . . . . .
I will show you fear in a handful of dust
[Eliot, "The Wasteland," 1922, pp. 53–54].

To search for one's parent and to find fear in a handful of dust: such a dilemma precipitates a hunger for visceral contact with the parent's traumatized self. There are times when visceral encounters seem most acute in the suffering body. And so, the child may seek the missing parental other through the infliction of bodily suffering (see also Kreegman, 1987). A gentle boy like James found his only initiative in acts of sexual molestation; as a good man, he passively witnessed a woman's rape. He is not the only child of genocide survivors in whom I have found such disturbing sexual secrets; I have known others who sought the absent parental object through sexual trespass. Here, grief is now multiplied by grief and by the renewal of terror. James is a son who seeks his absent mother and absent aunt in what Frankel (1998, discussing Ferenczi) calls "objectless sensation": a suffering body void of words and human comfort.

To seek the parent through the parent's pain: this is a recognition that genocidal annihilation was not an experience of the mind, but of the senses. Its memory was inscribed in the viscera, and must be known through the viscera (see also Krystal, 1988; Van der Kolk, 1996). In massive psychic trauma, the body functions as death's wordless scribe, encoding "region after region of nullity" (Eigen, 1996, p. 106) in bodily symptoms, acts, and sensations. To decode this bodily evidence, to bond with the survivor's state of infinite nullification, the child may attempt to meet his parent in the intimate specificity of bodily torment. Unwitting, this child knows that "the ego is ultimately derived from bodily sensations, chiefly from those that spring from the surface of the body" (Freud, 1923, pp. 26–27); he knows that the collapse of this ego was likewise located in bodily sensation. To find the parents' traumatized and *pretraumatized* selves, this son reaches into and beyond their bodily degradation.

Such bodily transmutations of absent memory are an attempt to substitute the fearful "something" of memory for the dreadful "no-thing" of death (Kierkegaard, 1937; Heidegger, 1962; Yalom, 1980). The dynamism of human existence is littered with mutual elaborations and confabulations of that which is absent from trauma narratives. Both benign and malignant bodily enactments engage the child/witness in an effort to make present that parental self which is absent. They are an attempt to provide, "a great relation . . . [which] throws a bridge from self-being to self-being across the abyss of dread of the universe" (Buber, 1923, p. 175). Benign enactments sustain a vision of the absent other as a potential self-being. In malignant enactments, the perpetrator senses that the other must be found and cannot be found, because death itself has already consumed her. "No one can take the other's death from him" (Heidegger, 1962, p. 284): in that truth, the bridge from self-being to self-being falls away.

## PAIN AND ITS SEDUCTION

To apprehend the reproductive cycle in which the perpetrator seeks the missing other through the renewal of suffering, it is necessary to define pain and to comprehend its condition. Besides pain itself, there are other aversive bodily states that reach the intolerable: starvation, cold, exhaustion, heat, invasive sexual sensation. When these states are inflicted by another, when the victim's agency is extinguished, and there is neither escape nor any possibility of human appeal, these states may be considered under the rubric of "pain." Indeed they often become pain, or accompany it.

Like loneliness, such experiences of pain often exist in trauma's "empty circle," urgent in the desire to be known, yet beyond the reach of human knowing. Where pain is inescapable, extremities of pain coalesce with extremities of fear; the self covets disappearance, and gratefully disappears. The mind dissociates and the body becomes thankfully insensate; the body faints, enters coma, or succumbs to death. Thus the suffering body self is a vanishing body self that cannot be seen, even in its encounter with the perpetrator. Like all bodily life and experience it is not knowable outside the matrix of human interaction, yet it continually escapes registration and symbolization (Harris, 1998). As Scarry (1985) notes, all pain (not just that of malignant trauma) is without meaning or interpersonal referent; it is void of meaning, and is not of or for anything. Pain, like other forms of nonlinguistic experience, is "inconsistent with reflection, can never enter reflective consciousness at all" (Stern, 1997, p. 114).

Pain is the most autistic and immediate of all human experiences, and yet it refuses the mutuality of empathic conduction. Even with the greatest effort to grasp another's pain, Scarry argues that the pain of another is

> Vaguely alarming yet unreal, laden with consequence yet evaporating before the mind . . . pain comes unsharably into our midst as at once that which cannot be denied and that which cannot be confirmed . . . to have great pain is to have certainty; to hear that another person has pain is to have doubt [Scarry, 1985, pp. 4–7].

The reality of another's pain eludes us, but it is also fascinating and alluring. If to have pain is to have certainty, then pain signifies a riveting being-in-the-present, a radical alertness in extremity. Pain is a paradox: although it defies mutual knowledge, although it seeks (and sometimes finds) its own dissociative disappearance, aversive sensation can appear as the absolute antagonist to alienated living.

Pain is inescapable; it is an unmediated experience in which every moment is acute. It is without self-consciousness: never ashamed in its nakedness, always raw in its presence, it is not concerned with persona and concealment. And it cannot be silent: pain screams and moans and writhes through the body. As such, the experience of pain is not dulled by those platitudes which are civilization. Pain is a reprieve from mediated experience. It cannot be coopted by language: in its visceral alertness, pain disrupts the torpor of "language rules" and denials. As such, it closes what Harris (1998) calls the hallowed split between word and deed; it forces denial to succumb to that absolute knowing that exists outside of linguistic knowledge. Whatever torture is called, whatever "principle" is used for its justification, the victim's body registers the elemental truth of violation.

If to witness pain is to experience doubt (as per Scarry, 1985), it may also be to experience an existential seduction. Through the veil of doubt, the witness encounters another for whom all doubt has been extinguished. In pain's ultimate moment, just before the suffering self disappears into oblivion, the tortured exists at the very apex of *full presence and full revelation*. Such a moment possesses an elemental allure: it is a breach in the wall of human insularity and isolation. It is this breach of human isolation that partly accounts for our pop culture of violence. The more family and culture alienate us from experiencing ourselves and others as *really real, really present, and really embodied*, the greater the seduction of human violence. And because the alertness of agony inevitably collapses into the inertia of disappearance, because coma, death, and dissociation render opaque that which has just been exquisitely revealed, the perpetrator may require the endless repetition of pain. And for the survivor-perpetrator, the awakening of torture and the disappearance of the torture victim comforts even as it frustrates. It reassures the survivor–perpetrator that it is possible to disappear from bodily extremity; it *is* the disappearance of the survivor who perpetually longs to disappear. But it is also an illusory encounter in the execution itself. This time, the survivor can watch, vigilant and alert, for the precise moment when the tortured shift from presence to absence. This time, the perpetrator imagines he will miss nothing, and so, finds mutuality in the area of solitude.

Thus, the renewal of bodily suffering seems to offer a unique resolution to the paradox of annihilation. For the survivor–perpetrator, pain is an indisputable force that insists on the presence of the other in the execution itself. And when the tortured evacuates himself and at last disappears, the survivor–perpetrator experiences an illusion of mutual linkage in the obscure moment of dying. And what of someone like James, not a survivor himself, but the child of survivors of genocide? Why should he, unlike most children of survivors, lose his empathic identification with the victim and live out a perpetrator–bystander enactment? Lonely in relation to missing parental selves, outraged and sexually stimulated by his fantasy of what they had done to survive, and loyal to the parental edict that he know their memories without being told, he closed the void in parental body through the re-creation of pain.

## JAMES: THE EMPATHY OF WITNESSING, THE CRUELTY OF WITNESSING

A woman who daily labored in exhaustion, his aunt was vigilant in the night. No drug regimen could insure her of sleep. And when his mother slept, she woke with screams. Sometimes, she cried, "No, no," and then there would be silence. A few times James rose from bed to comfort her, and found her panting, eyes washed with tears. At such times, she did not know him, nor he her. She was gone; he could give her nothing. They were strangers; he was frozen, he could not touch her. His father went on sleeping in the adjacent bed. Of these times, he and his father never spoke. Once, he found his aunt rocking his mother; they were crying as they embraced. He was told to go back to bed. He was told nothing. Later his aunt would not leave the television to comfort his mother. Soon, he too learned not to awaken.

Often, the next day his mother would shut herself in a closet. Sometimes, there were sobs. James would be careful, still, waiting. His father and aunt went to work. Eventually, his mother would emerge, subdued, and resume cooking and cleaning. He did not ask, she did not explain. The mother of the massacre and the aunt of the massacre: they could not tell their story. They dominated the family discourse and lived forever beyond it. His mother revealed herself as no one, and shadowed his existence.

Unconsciously, he has wondered: why were they still alive, while all the others were dead? Had they hidden, had they been passive, mute and unprotesting, as they witnessed their family's murder? Perhaps they were the almost-dead but not-dead: living voluptuous bodies, raped amidst corpses, forced into prostitution. His life was the theater of these inarticulate possibilities. In the absence of their story, he lived their violation and submission; their terrorized, inert surrender was the leitmotif of his existence. Throughout most of his life, he experienced himself as bullied, invaded, and dominated. He had no interior but that which was violated and stolen. The others in his work world were envisioned as vast in stature, violent, and armored with infinite, annihilating power. He was without shelter or recourse. At the possibility of assertion, his heart raced, his hands shook, and sweat ran; his mind was blank, and he was bereft of all words. It was as if he felt: *If I am angry they will surely kill me; if I submit, I may be left alive. And that life that I am left to live will be an impoverished bodily degradation, shadowed by longing and remembrance.*

Always poised for a moment of flight, he hides food, clothes, and money; he has secrets he confides to no one. His wife has longed to know him, they are amicable, and yet he maintains his silence. His children complain that he overprotected them. He cares for his grandchildren with tenderness and vigilant terror, awaiting the day when he will impotently witness their destruction. He will have survived them from his hiding place; he will fail as their rescuer, and will survive them through his betrayal of his beloved. He has lived these primordial fantasies for 65 years, never associating it with the Armenian genocide.

In treatment, we had studied the gap between James's dream image and the scream. Through this gap, through his ordinary conversation, genocide grew in its story and precipitated the awakening of a sexualized transference. It was here that I discovered the analogue to rape. Sometimes he *is* that deadened nerve which the raped woman aspires to become. And sometimes, he *acts* on the skin surface of a woman to evoke his aunt and his mother in their visceral torment. As he acts on a woman's body, he evokes the presence of his relatives' perpetrators, placing solitude in human interaction, converting torment to mastery, converting absence to presence.

He had always been sexually preoccupied. He began to tell me his sexual fantasies in intimate and scarifying detail. My body was entered into them: I was seduced, humiliated, bought, and sold. He wondered if he aroused me, and he wondered this with glee. What began under the guise of an analytic excavation became an invasive assault on my body. He did not want to find the meaning of his fantasies, he wanted a shared erotic elaboration of them. He knew we couldn't have *actual* sex. But in his manner of telling me *about* sex, he was attempting to have it with me. He was not desirous of excavating meaning. He was desirous of erotic degradation. He would not lie down, but faced me, scrutinizing my features, delighting in my blush, in the bodily manifestations of my discomfort. Always, he had been so kindhearted; now, he was engaged in a practiced attack on my viscera. He would seem alternately sadistic and playful, sometimes empathically responsive to my discomfort. Eventually, I stopped him. I decided that he would not be permitted to so discomfort me; he was not to be permitted to have sex through sex talk.

There was an empathic James, an I–Thou James, a timid man of great tenderness and compassion. But in the bodily transference enactment, we found another James, whose memories were dim and barely remembered. For him, women's bodies were an "it": soft, erotic commodities to be bought, stolen, or sold. This James was the perpetrator-bystander, enacting and facilitating the violation of women. In stopping this James from trespass, I finally heard his memories.

At the age of 30, he had been coming home late at night through a city park when he heard a woman screaming and moaning. He crept forward in the shelter of some trees. In the shadows he witnessed a woman being held down by two men. Terrified, immobilized, fascinated, he watched as they beat her about her face and took turns raping her. He remembered initial confusion: were these dim shapes two men and a woman? Was this a portrait of violence or of union? Were they going to rape her or merely rob her? Through this paralysis, he was aware of a vague sense that he should run for the police; then he felt terrified that the rapists would attack him. He remembered being aroused. He did nothing.

Eventually, the woman stopped screaming and stopped struggling; she lay inert beneath the trees. The men finished with her, and left. James emerged from his daze, and left his hiding place, without approaching the woman or offering her aid. He did not know if she was alive. He went home the way he had come, telling no one, fearful of getting "involved." Over the next few months, he occasionally found himself wondering if she had survived; intermittently he felt deep shame, and then the incident vanished. He had never shared this experience with anyone, and it had fallen into complete disappearance, until the memory was reawakened in the sexualization of my body.

This story eventually led to the telling of another, also shocking, but this time, oddly void of all shame. It began when he was age 10. He always remembered being sexually stimulated, frustrated and desirous. He stole "peeps" at women's breasts, stared through neighbors' windows as they undressed. Sometimes they caught him, and he got in trouble. He pursued glimpses of his aunt and his mother: through doors left barely ajar, as they bent over at the stove, as they stood above him on the stairs. Beginning in puberty, he had an intense sexual fantasy life: alternately, either he or the woman was humiliated, exploited, betrayed, aroused. As he moved into puberty and adolescence, his sense of desire and frustration heightened, as did his paralytic loneliness. He was too shy to initiate contact with girls. At the young age of 17, he despaired of sex with his peers. Then he thought of his mother and his aunt: their bodies had always nurtured him, comforted him. Why should they not comfort him in this new bodily urgency and desolation?

With virtually no anxiety or shame or reflection, he embarked on a premeditated plan to initiate sex with either his aunt or his mother. Both his aunt and his mother had always come to him at night when he had migraines, never recognizing that the child had become a man. One of them would come again. He pretended to have a migraine. This time it was his aunt who came to him; as always, she put her arm around him, caressed his head, and lay still in his bed. He began to caress her breasts through her nightgown, imagining her arousal, or at least, her compliance. She did not move; he felt her body go limp with resignation. With great sadness, she said in Armenian, "You are like my son. You do this to a mother?" He removed his hand. After a few minutes of silence, she left his bed. They never spoke of this incident; it too fell away into disappearance. But neither she nor his mother ever entered his bed again.

He told this story with a mild embarassment and did not consider it incest. I wondered where his shame and guilt were; I wondered if she had not sexually seduced and violated him prior to this incident. How did an acutely empathic, lonely, and passive boy find his only initiative in the molestation of his own aunt? How were the sexual boundaries lost? And more particularly: how had his beloved aunt become an object of exploitation? All the usual lines of inquiry failed to entirely elucidate this mystery. Yes, his father had been a cipher; his mother and his aunt were his only parental objects. She and his mother had entered his bed for many years, overstimulating him certainly, but they only placed their arms around him. Their nightgowns were not filmy negligees, but flannel; their figures were not voluptuous, but matronly and concealed. They smelled, not of perfume, but of sweat and bread baking. He had no memories of having been molested or prematurely sexualized. He had been aroused by his *fantasy* of their bodies, imagining them as young, firm, voluptuous. But he *knew* their plump bodies as "mama." Yes, the women were closer to him than to his father; he had no siblings and one could say he was a two-time oedipal winner. But none of this accounted for his lapse in human empathy, for his sudden emergence into agency. It was then that we began to inquire how he imagined they had survived. He began to speak of his lifelong conviction that they had complied with rape and with prostitution.

When speaking of his nightmares, of the gap between the image and the scream, James and I had met his mother and aunt at the brink of the massacre: there was ordinary life, and then there were families ripped asunder, screams, blows, the first rivulets of blood, and then there was nothing. We would meet them again, on the other side: wandering in displaced person camps, dazed, then a boat to America, poverty and dislocation. Another gap, and then the renewed ordinariness of living, and the eventual eruption of the scream. We never met them in the moments of their relatives' murder, in their presumptive rape, in an ongoing life lived in brutal excoriation. Our minds inevitably collapsed and went blank: what he lived possessed no image, no words, no memory, although he now knew he was living that which he had never been told. Although his waking and dream life proliferated with images of genocidal violation, still his night terrors (fewer now) persisted: the pedestrian event, the blank, and then the scream. He read histories of the Turkish genocide. He searched faded letters written from Armenia, finding cryptic references to three dead brothers, to a decimated village, to dispersed friends, to unwanted children born of the enemy. Were some of these children his own stepbrothers, stepsisters, cousins? Had his aunt or mother abandoned a despised child? There was no one left to ask; the authors of the letters were long dead.

But the James who molested his aunt was the child of women whom he both hated and longed for. They were women who lived in a continual state of disappearance: disappearing into young girls enduring genocide, disappearing into young girls enduring rape, vanishing into the Turks' willing harlots. He is the child of region after region of nullity, falling endlessly through space, alone and uncontained. He hates these young girls for their absence and longs for their reappearance. He imagines them as *present* in their perpetrators' beds. When his mother is sealed in the closet, he is without her, and so he enters the closet by becoming her persecutory object: now she can never shut him out. Indeed, his aunt might even embrace his advances. Perhaps the woman who is raped in the park seeks this union with her rapists.

He is like the child who "might have perceived his protecting object not to be able to indemnify him against terror but rather to reify and confirm its full horror" (Grotstein, 1979, p. 436). How much has he hated those young girls in Armenia who continually steal his mother and his aunt from him? How much has he blamed them for his timidity, for the insularity of an immigrant life alienated from his peers? Often he has needed those innocent, joyful young girls to be present for *him* and not for the Turks. Surely, they might have shown him another world, a world of confidence, of play, of all kinds of adventure. But when he reaches for these young girls, he finds shadowy harlots of death occupying the maternal body, providing maternal bodily functions. Perhaps he has identified with those who stole their bodies from them. Has he not a right to this theft? His empathic self has starved for them, imbibed their fear for them, and tried to secure them against disaster. And yet, he still finds them absent and himself empty. Why not mirror his father's willful blindness to their pain? In his molestation of his aunt, in his passive witnessing of a stranger's rape, James resurrects the absent mother of genocide. He meets a raped young girl, violated with no right of refusal, stripped of her subjectivity. And in the moment of his aunt's violation, he restores that young girl's grief, and empowers her refusal in the removal of his hand. In excavating the memory of a raped woman's body lying inert in the park, he comes to understand that young girls hiding from massacre do not invite a murderer's sexual embrace. Since the first moments of the slaughter, those young girls have been present for no one.

And what of his aunt, passive and resigned. Perhaps she thought of her nephew/son as her remaining link to that which is human: he was the only male whom she might touch without imminent violation. Her brother-in-law she does not touch. In the course of James's analysis, he came to suspect that his father might have attempted sex with his aunt at one time, causing her distance from the father and exacerbating her nightly vigilance. Every other man of import has either raped her or died. But she imagines this: that of all human codes, the incest taboo is sacred, inviolable. Surely here she might entrust her body, find and give comfort and tenderness, perhaps even finding sleep. Is she tempting James, testing him as she enters his bed, longing to find the restitution of innocence in the boy who becomes a man? Is she transmitting that which cannot be communicated: an unspeakable rape resurrected through incestuous victimization? Or perhaps, as he screams in the night, she hears her brothers, her father; perhaps she comforts him as she was prohibited from comforting their dying bodies. Entering his bed throughout his adolescence, she has collapsed him into her fantasy, and into her longing, and has refused to know him as an autonomous evolving sexual adult.

In the incestuous enactment he has almost met his mothers in the execution itself. They had shared his adolescent bed in a condition of forgetfulness; now his aunt emerges from that bed in a state of mournful awakening. She had met his incestuous gesture in a condition of anguish and submissive despair: absolutely knowing and largely resigned, a woman who knew no possibility of refusal. And yet, she had ventured a tentative refusal: "You are like my son. You do this to a mother?" Together, James and his aunt moved in and out of dissociative contagion, representing the rape that lived at the vortex of her "empty circle," then returning it in silence. He was her perpetrator; she was his "it," he had felt nothing for her, and had refused to remember. But he had healed her in the removal of his hand.

## PSYCHOANALYSIS AND THE PERSISTENCE OF BODY EVIDENCE

Because trauma is "written on the body" (see McDougall, 1989; Herman, 1992; Van der Kolk, 1996) we must listen for its repetition in the analytic body. In this way, we do not "graft speech onto silence" (Langer, 1995, p. 20), but rather illuminate silence and render it audible. Through her own bodily sensation, the analyst encounters pain's contradictions: its condition of autistic certainty and interpersonal doubt; the way being-present meets the prospect of total disappearance. We can understand the way bodily pain locates the other "who could have and should have been there," the other who will be forever absent, engulfed in the "infinite nullification" of the execution.

As analysts treating the problems of evil, we cannot conceive of the treatment of trauma as a path moving toward an emotionally integrated, linguistically encoded story in which bodily symptoms heal through their narration. To view traumatic healing as a progressive movement from the nonlinguistic to the linguistic, from fragmentation to cohesion, and from solitude to mutuality is to suffer from an excess of hope. Such hope imagines that the traumatized self can finally locate the other who should have been there, and in that meeting, death itself will be defeated. But analysis is not larger than death, and it is not larger than the solitude of survival. Indeed, Freud (1937) cautions us not to behave as though "it were possible by means of analysis to attain to a level of absolute psychical normality . . . as though we had succeeded in resolving every one of the patient's repressions and in *filling in all the gaps in his memory*" (pp. 219–220; italics added).

Just as we think we have rendered bodily states and enactments in a complete trauma narrative, just as we seem to have freed the patient's body from repetition, the evidence carried in our patient's body reasserts itself. Whether we treat evil's victim, its bystander, or its perpetrator, bodily evidence remains as the living testimonial of the damned. It articulates the outer limits of human connection and the evolving linguistic narrative. This tension serves as a history of the execution; although it can never be fully liberated and transformed in to language, neither can it be bound and eviscerated by a dominant discourse. What the tongue cannot speak and what reason cannot comprehend, what is absolutely certain and absolutely in doubt: this is the relational nexus of evil. The analyst must remember that, for this patient, "words themselves feel more or less meaningless. The person carries a sense of internal isolation as his natural state, and trying to convey this in words is experienced as an exercise in futility. . . . In the interplay of silence and words, a patient can, at least potentially, force the analyst to give up his attempt to 'understand' his patient and allow himself to 'know' his patient" (Bromberg, 1994, p. 524). Only if the patient–therapist dyad continues to be moved by the "limited power of words to release the specific kinds of physical distress haunting the caverns of deep memory" (Langer, 1991, p. 8) can we move closer to arresting evil's reproduction. Only then will the autism of bodily pain be transmuted into mourning. In this mourning, the body continues speaking, pursuing meaning, and asserting itself in the dissolution of meaning.

As analysts, we must accept that the pathway toward healing is a dialectic, in which the press toward the healing narrative evocation of memory is continuously countered by the visceral resurrection of that which is beyond human encounter. Here, the imperative to tell continually meets the impossibility of telling; new words are always found and are always found insufficient. Mutuality collapses into solitude, and then solitude reaches for mutuality. Language will always obfuscate all that it illuminates (Schachtel, 1959; Price, 1995; Harris 1996; Grand, 1997c; Shapiro, 1997; Bromberg, 1998). We must not elevate the power of language. It is through the body's disorganization of language and reason that we derive the lived sense that "the force of this (traumatic) experience would appear to arise precisely . . . in the collapse of its understanding" (Caruth, 1995, p. 7). For, as Dimen (1998) suggests, body matters are often the antagonist of language: "Enactment and embodiment have in common their habitation of the inarticulate" (p. 66). When remorse and human mourning awaken from the depths of human evil, they will continually reveal themselves in the very *limits* of human communion, in the inarticulate loneliness of the body.

## JAMES: MOURNING AND THE PERSISTENCE OF BODY EVIDENCE

At last, in his analysis, he realized the body he had molested was the body of his beloved aunt, the woman who had comforted and nourished him, despite being haunted by memory. He remembered now her hopeless protest, her resignation, the infinite sadness in her voice; he remembered feeling a tear coursing down her cheek as he removed his hand. He remembered the anonymous woman whose rape he had witnessed, and whom he had not rescued. She has haunted him in his dreams. He weeps, and feels there can be no end to this weeping.

He could not break their silence, he could make no reparation, offer them no comfort. He was limited by the passage of time, by the finality of their deaths. The night terrors lessened, continued, and changed shape. The narrative of his life, and the narrative of his relatives' rape grew and disappeared: he knew both more and less, and became both more and less lonely. He felt undeserving of a life without culpability. It was this awakening that deepened and enriched his own loneliness. Suddenly impotent where he had always been obsessively sexual, his body self embraced its penance, and its despair. His wife's body reminded him of his aunt's at the time of the molestation. Her breasts were his aunt's breasts; he could no longer "assault" them. His wife said to him that he was really talking for the first time in 40 years, that he was more affectionate as well. She wonders about his loss of desire, but is also freed from his compulsive pursuit of sex. He could not tell her about the nature of his impotence. He knows that there was a place inside of him to which he could not take her. His sexual dysfunction is an area of solitude, to be shared only with the dead. Refusing analytic and medical intervention, he despairs, and yet, he considers himself healed. He does not want to eradicate his body's testimonial. He calls me periodically, when he feels an excess of loneliness. In the periodic encounter with another who knows what is inscribed on his body, he searches for two young girls disappearing into genocide. And together we know that they will never be found.

> If the lost word is lost, if the spent word is spent
> . . . . . . . .
> Where shall the word be found, where will the word
> Resound? Not here, there is not enough silence
> Not on the sea or on the islands, not
> On the mainland, in the desert or the rain land
> For those who walk in darkness
> Both in the day time and in the night time
> The right time and the right place are not here
> [Eliot, "Ash Wednesday," 1922, p. 92].

# CHAPTER 3

# CHILD ABUSE AND THE PROBLEM
# OF KNOWING HISTORY

❧

IN THE PERPETRATION OF EVIL, in the elaboration of the execution itself, there is always another story. In this story, truth and illusion, memory and imagination exist in a mutual commentary. If what stories can do is make things present (O'Brian, 1990), if the execution itself is always absent, then stories are told to register a truth that cannot be found in the simple telling of facts. For, as O'Brian (1990) suggests, "In war, you lose your sense of the definite, hence your sense of truth itself, and therefore it's safe to say that in a true war story nothing is absolutely true" (p. 88). As Alpert (1997) has suggested, the authentic rendering of annihilation may require that lies, confabulations, and imaginative elaborations carry truths, and that truths carry lies. In this labyrinth, the victim is at the mercy of our listening. We must listen, and prepare to be bewildered; we must be bewildered and yet persist in the pursuit of historical truth. For in the arena of the really *real*, war is being fought, a child is being beaten. As clinicians treating the problem of evil, we must seek a pathway toward truth that registers both the *impossibility* of knowing history and the *imperative* to know history. We must be steadfast in the conviction that there is a "movement, however torturous, from ignorance to knowledge, from mythical thought and childish fantasies to perception of reality face to face, to knowledge of true goals, true values as well as truths of fact" (Berlin, 1991, p. 7), even as we know that what really happened, happened in obscurity.

## THE PROBLEM OF TRUTH IN THE PSYCHOANALYSIS OF EVIL

We psychoanalysts are practicing in a paradoxical historical moment that is full of extraordinary contradiction and exciting potential. We are developing a view of the analytic situation as a rich field of relational play: a world of mutually constructed meanings and intersubjective truths. These truths are explored in an egalitarian, two-person relationship in which, at long last, the patient is permitted to "see and know" the analyst, to have and possess his or her own perceptions of the analytic reality, and to "negotiate" (Pizer, 1999) that reality with the analyst. At the very moment we relinquish the pursuit of historical truth, however, we are simultaneously attempting to integrate trauma theory and research into psychoanalysis (Alpert, 1994; Davies and Frawley, 1994). But here we have a contradiction and a conundrum: the treatment of all trauma is predicated on a shared conviction between analyst and patient that the trauma actually occurred. The establishment of the actual historicity of trauma is particularly necessary with child abuse. Child abuse is a trauma uniquely characterized by the falsification of reality; it has invariably occurred secretly, in family systems that deny its very existence. Survivors of other forms of malignant trauma, such as war or violent crime, all receive the profound support of consensual validation from survivor cohorts and the larger culture. The child abuse survivor (particularly the incest survivor) has been robbed of reality and of history; cure requires its restoration.

Unlike the one-person, classic, archaeological model, the new social constructivism releases the incest/child abuse survivor to repossess her own perceptions and experiences, rather than to defer the definition of perception to authority/analyst/parent. This repossession is vital to her recovery. However, she finds herself once again lost in funhouse mirrors if she seeks to resolve the historical reality of her ambiguous, dissociated memories in an analysis operating on this constructivist model. While there is endless empathic space for analyst and patient to "converse," as Spezzano (1993) says, about the patient's desire for historical truth, the actual facts of trauma would be considered inaccessible, lost forever in what Spence (1982, 1993) describes as the endless embellishments and distortions of language, time, and memory. This only leaves us with that analytic vista that Geha (1993) calls the fictions of the mind: "[M]ind-made realities constitute for human beings their sole realms of existence, and that it is only about these realms that anything at all can be known. No other knowable realities exist"(p. 209).

In such moments, psychoanalysis appears to border on a relativism that is bankrupt with regard to real evil. At other moments, what Aron (1996) describes as a moderate, affirmative postmodern position is proposed: here authors such as Hoffman (1992), Mitchell (1993b, 1995), Gill (1995), Aron (1996), Clarke (1997), and others subscribe to the vision of external reality proposed by Gill (1995): "A construction is subject to the constraints of reality even if we cannot say what the reality is" (p. 2). Here, as Aron (1996) notes, relativism is constrained by an external reality, but "what we understand of reality is only a construction of reality" (p. 29). In this perspective, there is nevertheless an interest in discriminating between "what is true and what is not" (Clarke, 1997, p. 11), an interest that Mitchell (1993b) suggests we pursue through careful contextual analysis and disciplined reason.

For psychoanalysts to refuse the reproduction of evil, we must immerse ourselves in the contradictions of narration and history, insisting on the immanence of historical truth, knowing that the history of annihilation undergoes continuous occlusion. The analyst must sustain a view of history as immutable and knowable, interpretable and subjective, both real and imagined. This position would hold both the objective and subjective components of truth (Hanly, 1995; Gabbard, 1997) and allow us to return to an awareness of what Sampson (1992) calls a person's innate, primary, and powerful interest in reality. For as Sass (1993) says, "It is the patient's life that is at stake, and the sheer undeniable reality of his or her emotions and memories may well make the patient less than enthusiastic about the prospect of engaging in some kind of aestheticist or deconstructive game" (p. 251). In the context of the malignant use of another, in the high stakes game of malignant dissociative contagion, it becomes ever more urgent to hold the hard objective edge of human history. If we find it difficult to hold onto the existence of this objective hard edge in the midst of our narrative investigations, we can renew our conviction through the research on traumatic memory. Herman and Harvey (1993) and Van der Kolk (1996), for example, have ascertained that memory traces are registered physiologically and motorically, although they are frequently dissociated. While traumatic memory does not exist in the linear verbal form in which we retain nontraumatic memory; while it is sensory, pictorial and enacted through a consistent constellation of posttraumatic stress disorder (PTSD) symptoms and signs, historical truth *exists*, written on the body.

With our adult patients, we must neither remain in the pure realm of subjectivity and interpretation nor imagine that the patient's story (or traumatic symptom picture) represents simple veridical memory. We must not foreclose *either* historical truth *or* the meaning of confabulations, fantasies, and distortions. How hard it has been for analysts to remain in that realm between certainty and doubt, where evil locates the contradictions of its history. How hard, and yet, how imperative: for evil will find its permit in the foreclosure of either form of truth, the narrative or the historic.

## *1984:* THE ANNIHILATION OF HISTORY AND SUBJECTIVITY

George Orwell's *1984* is a tale of oppression and of the annihilation of human subjectivity. It satires the extreme consequences of constructivism; of the dangers of pursuing only narrative truth, where this "truth" is transacted in a culture of evil.

Oceania is a bleak and merciless totalitarian state in which the human soul is on the verge of extinction. Thought and subjectivity are legislated; hatred flourishes, love is punishable by death. All human bonds are forbidden. Even as Big Brother annihilates one's soul, he is experienced as the sole parental protector, the only beloved.

In this dark place, Winston is the singular man who has retained his soul; he lives in an agony of loneliness and despair. He is an old-fashioned existential man; he is not a constructivist. He believes in the immutability of history, of memory, and of truth. He knows that in a world of oppression, one cannot compromise on the truth: there are only truths and lies. One must hold onto memory and truth because without memory there is no interiority, a condition for the integrity of the human soul. He knows, as Sass (1993) says, that "to experience the more intense and full-blooded emotions—love and hate, sadness and simple joy—may require a sense of existential rootedness that is inconsistent with radical fictionalism; namely a grounding in the lived-body, feelings of connection with solid objects and living human beings, and an awareness of finitude of finality and of risk" (p. 252). Like the child abuse or incest survivor, this very knowledge places Winston at risk for terrible retribution. Winston works in the Ministry of Truth, where all recorded history is rewritten daily in accordance with the latest Party lie, so that there will never be any documentary evidence about "what really happened." Doublethink is practiced so that the workers in the ministry know and don't know that history has been altered: they are able to know they are lying and yet believe the lie seamlessly. Winston alone grasps the enormous implications of the destruction of history: "If the party could thrust its hand into the past and say of this or that even it never happened—that surely was more terrifying than mere torture and death" (Orwell, 1949, p. 33). Winston understands that with torture and death, the human soul may remain alive, but the annihilation of one's history and of one's capacity to know reality results in what Shengold (1989) calls "soul murder." Where history and memory are completely mutable and in the hands of one's oppressor, one is emptied of will, autonomy, and humanity. Even as Winston is desperately trying to retain his memory of history, while he attempts to locate any source of evidence that history is not what the Party says it is, he finds himself lost in the ambiguous fog of memory that characterizes the incest survivor: "The past, he reflected, has not merely been altered, it had been actually destroyed . . . everything melted into mist. Sometimes, indeed you could put your finger on a definite lie, but you could prove nothing. There was never any evidence" (p. 33).

Winston has received the early recognition of his loving mother, and so, unlike the child abuse survivor, he is capable of knowing the truth in complete solitude, but he cannot bear the agony of living a false life without ever having been known. Risking arrest and death, he forms two relationships of love: one with Julia and one with O'Brian. With Julia he shares an exquisite rebellion of private sensuality, tenderness, and warmth. But he cannot share his concern about the eradication of history and memory with her; she is not interested and doesn't understand its significance; when he speaks of it, she falls asleep. Because of this disinterest, her subjectivity seems limited, ephemeral, and transient; ultimately he cannot be fully known by her. (In a sense, this is a metaphor for the fatal flaw of the social-constructivist context for psychoanalysis: it provides a vibrant field in which to experience one's aliveness, but it is unconscious with regard to the importance of actual memory.) This is the fatal flaw in Winston's relationship to Julia, which drives him into the arms of inner party member O'Brian.

For many years, Winston and O'Brian have studied each other without speaking. In O'Brian's face Winston perceives his soulmate: a deeply intelligent man, full of compassion and suffering, secretly antagonistic to the party and the only living person with whom Winston can share his concern about the immutability of memory. In Winston's deep longing to be known, he gradually relinquishes his vigilant knowledge that O'Brian is a dangerous inner party member, much as the abused child idealizes her parent and denies what she knows. Winston persuades Julia that they should reveal themselves to O'Brian in the hope that O'Brian will connect them with the underground; and for one extraordinary moment this escape indeed seems possible. Knowing that they may be arrested at any time, Winston and Julia agree that although they will undoubtedly say anything under torture, it will not constitute a betrayal of one another unless they stop loving one another. This betrayal they believe to be impossible, for how can anyone get inside of you like that? The next day, Winston and Julia are arrested and Winston discovers that O'Brian is his personal torturer and interrogator. So begins Winston's most intimate relationship, one in which he is completely known and completely violated: tortured, comforted, understood, and annihilated. These are the moments of incest. O'Brian remains awake and engaged during Winston's courageous discourses about history; he very much shares Winston's conviction that without immutable history there is no survival of the human soul. Winston can endure tremendous pain and abuse without losing himself, because the pain is inflicted by his beloved, who recognizes him fully even though he tortures him. But Winston is seeking mutuality; O'Brian is seeking dominance and power. Winston cherishes the immutability of memory because it makes him human; O'Brian must destroy it. Like the incestuous parent, O'Brian knows he will only gain absolute power when he has eradicated Winston's autonomous conviction about memory, when he has seduced and terrorized Winston into willing surrender of both his subjectivity and his history. The seduction of Winston's soul and his voluntary submission to a falsified reality is achieved through the simultaneous promise of exquisite recognition and the threat of annihilation terror; this process precisely replicates the dynamic of incest and childhood physical abuse. Mere pain is inadequate; O'Brian takes Winston into Room 101, where he meets his greatest terror: carnivorous rats. Winston can survive starvation and brutality; he does not fear death; but here he is subjected to disintegration anxiety. In a desperate effort to avoid the rats, he cries out: Do it to Julia. He feels it—he wishes they would do it to her instead. In the same moment he has betrayed Julia and lost her he has relinquished his soul forever. He is empty and can be filled with the Party's lies and love of Big Brother. Once O'Brian has successfully broken Winston, dissolved his resistance and his memory, the bond between them ends much as the perpetrator's interest in the child would dissolve if the child were a dead thing, incapable of human response, of sexuality, of fear and resistance. Winston can no longer offer O'Brian the recognition that O'Brian has coerced from him. Winston retains only the memory of his own betrayal of himself and of Julia in Room 101; he cannot remember the long chain of abuse; he loves Big Brother. Indeed, O'Brian has gotten inside him in ways Winston had never believed possible, but which O'Brian had predicted: "Things will happen to you from which you could not recover, if you lived a thousand years never again will you be capable of ordinary human feeling. Everything will be dead inside you. Never again will you be capable of love, or friendship or joy of living, or laughter, or curiosity or courage or integrity. You will be hollow. We shall squeeze you empty and then we shall fill you with ourselves" (p. 211). The abuse survivor has indeed been squeezed empty, and is filled only with the perpetrator. But unlike the annihilated Winston, the survivor may sustain a buried wish to be recognized and to have her history and subjectivity restored. She will seek that restoration in the unique properties of the analyst's listening. The analyst's capacity to witness both certainty and doubt and to grasp both historic and narrative truths enables the patient to experience the history of the execution itself. And in the analyst's pursuit of *what really happened*, a real victim may be rescued from a real evil.

## BOB: WHEN LIES CARRY TRUTHS, AND TRUTHS CARRY LIES

These are times when knowing history seems like an imperative. At these times, locating history often seems like an impossibility. And yet, we must persist in the conviction that fact and fiction take up joint residence in our patient's material.

Bob was a compulsive liar, brought to treatment at the age of fifteen. He was depressed, dysfunctional, unable to eat. It was as if he were in mourning, but there was no one apparent for him to mourn. His parents brought him reluctantly. Prior to meeting Bob, I met his mother and his father, now divorced and remarried to new spouses, both of whom refused to meet me. Together, the mother and the father told their own story: a decent family, marital stress and alienation, mother's secret affair, father's discovery of it, their divorce when Bob was ten. The mother recalled Bob being more troubled by the divorce than his older sister, but that had passed. I asked if Bob could have known about the mother's affair? No, it was well concealed. Had the father had affairs? No, never. There were no traumas. Both parents agreed that Bob was difficult, contrary, withdrawn, and a compulsive liar. Among several more pedestrian examples, the father told a disturbing story: that Bob had told a friend that his father had been beating him. This story was presented compellingly, as evidence of a lie among lies.

Then I met Bob and began seeking and losing the truth carried by his lies. Depressed, desolate, and solitary, he lived in the anticipation of abandonment. He told me two secrets. One was a secret I must keep for him: his stepfather beat his mother, and Bob had been forbidden to tell me (or anyone). Intimidated by his new stepfather, he was disturbed by his inability to protect his mother. He claimed that if the mother knew I knew, she would remove him from treatment. Bob said nothing of being abused by the father, or by the stepfather, or of ever having been the victim of abuse. I believed him. But then, there was the confession of his lies.

It was not a small, insignificant lie, but one of vast and malignant proportions. It exploited friends, family, teachers, counselors, and it may have precipitated more than one death. For one year he had embellished this lie, knowing it was a lie, and yet believing it seamlessly. In some way the lie was more true than any other real experience. But he was desirous of release from the daily convolutions of omissions, evasions, truths, half-truths. Anticipating the wholesale retribution that would attend his confession, his depression seemed linked to the imminence of loss.

And so, he told me the lie. Like all lies it began with some truths, and some understandable evasions. For about two years, he had been attracted by boys. Briefly, he had been "seeing" a boy from another school, and had fallen in love. Intentionally ambiguous about the lover's gender, he had told friends of his new relationship. Allowing them to think that the boy was a girl, he spoke about his love. And then the boy broke off with him, and he was left with a layered humiliation: the secret that the girl was a boy, the secret that he had been seduced and rejected. Shame was unbearable. He continued to tell peers of dates and intimate exchanges with the "girlfriend," never revealing that it had been a brief homosexual encounter. Over the next two months, an ever-expanding circle of friends and teachers came to know of this passionate love, and yet no one had met this Romeo's Juliet. Bob would absent himself for ostensible "dates," wandering bleakly through parks until curfew, returning cold and desolate from his "assignations." Friends wanted to meet her, but he claimed he had to keep their relation a secret because she was older, and of another race: their parents would not abide their relationship. He refused to even reveal her name. Thus this modest, retiring boy became the subject of intrigue, a romantic of great and tragic mystery.

His lies began to strain others' credulity; friends began to wonder aloud if there was something "wrong." Increasingly alienated from his actual relationships, having his most significant relationship with a phantom, it occurred to Bob that if his love was "dead," there would be an end to lies. And so he "killed her off" in a drunk driving accident over a weekend. Pointing to an article in a local newspaper about a drunk driving accident in another town, he at last "identified" the girlfriend. Bob had no difficulty simulating mourning. He had been mourning since the boy had cut Bob off; he had been mourning for the collapse of his authenticity since the beginning of his lies. During the pretense of a fulfilled joyful connection, Bob had concealed depression; now he had only to reveal it. He wept, he lost weight, failed to concentrate in school, and spoke endlessly of loss. As he continued in his fabrication, he felt a resurgence of authenticity and connection. Friends were devoted, compassionate, and generous toward him in his grief. Then, in their concern they sought advice and counsel from their teachers, counselors, and parents.

The tragic aspect of the girl's death inspired anxiety in the adults in Bob's school community: they were already worried about drunk driving. Although Bob's parents never seemed to know what was going on, teachers, counselors, and the referring school psychologist were concerned. Previously a cipher at home and at school, Bob was now the focus of attention. He told increasingly elaborate stories about sneaking into the funeral (their love had to remain secret, as always), about witnessing the grief of her family and friends. Eventually, school authorities exhorted Bob to address an assembly of his peers about drunk driving. He spoke about his loss, argued passionately against drunk driving, became a tragic hero. In the first weeks of therapy, however, the thread began to unravel, and someone at the school discovered he was lying. Within weeks, the entire school knew of it and repudiated him. Teenagers whom he had previously inspired toward sobriety became ever more cynical and ever more drunk, until real drunk-driving accidents occurred. Somewhat reasonably, he felt that he had potentiated these deaths with his flagrant hypocrisy. Once a tragic hero, he was now contemptible. Once comforted by an extensive support network, he was now ostracized.

This false construction seemed to carry some truth that had to be packaged in lies. But what was it, and why was it carried by lies? What was this grief, this humiliation: who was the "secret" man who "seduced" and abandoned? Who was the dead, and who was his "killer"? Bob was too young for such metaphorical inquiry; instead we spoke of his difficulty accepting and revealing his homosexuality. And we spoke of truth and of lies. And then, there were other stories. Of course, he had always known that his mother had an affair—he had read letters, overheard conversations. Of course, his father had affairs. And he was a daily witness to his mother's deferential lies to the stepfather, lies designed to forestall violent explosions. He quickly grasped the family subtext: the unconscious prescription to lie, the manifest proscription against lying. Apparently he was considered the family's "bad" liar; to be a "good" liar was this family's equivalent of an "honest man." Bob became committed to telling the truth, and struggled nobly in his relationships to work through the damage he had done. He "came out" to family and friends. Already ridiculing him, many reviled him. But a few new friendships emerged. Gradually, he reestablished some equilibrium, began to eat, to function in school, to emerge from despair. His parents were satisfied that the depression was "cured," but they were not pleased at his homosexuality, and hoped that it was a "phase" that could likewise be cured. I worked to support his self-esteem and self-conviction, and to help them love their son in his real identity.

But what really did it all mean, and did I now have the true story? One day his school called. A gym teacher had discovered fresh burn marks on Bob's back. According to Bob, he had leaned against a candelabrum. Knowing him to be a liar, and finding the explanation absurd, the teacher approached the school counselor, who called the parents. The school nurse said the burns looked like they had been made with a cigarette. A friend remembered being told that the father was abusive. Social agencies were called. The parents were credible in their denial. Bob held to his story. But we all knew he was a liar. When he next came to see me, I asked to see the burns. There were four neat burns in the middle of his back. Monosyllabic, minimizing his pain, he would tell me nothing different from his prepared story. The school had gotten hysterical, his parents had done nothing. I said I knew he was a liar. I said his stepfather beat his mother. He said that was true, but that he had never touched Bob. I asked if there was someone else in his life who might have burned him. He said no. I suggested he might be afraid to tell the truth. He insisted that he only told the truth now. I wondered if the burns were parental retribution for his homosexuality, or perhaps the result of homophobic violence at school. His story was unassailable, the burns healed and turned to scars. The school and social service agencies had to wait and assess further incidents. We all knew that in this family, everyone was credible, and everybody lied. Shortly after, he left for summer camp. His parents, satisfied with his "progress" and fearful of further accusations, refused to continue his treatment. They have failed to respond to follow-up calls, and the school has failed to pinpoint the source of the abuse.

## HISTORICAL TRUTH AND IMAGINATIVE MEMORY

In the prism of tall tales, burns exist indisputably on a boy's back. These burns bear the hard objective edge of history. And while their "truth" is incontestable, their meaning is encoded in fantasy and confabulation. In his tale of a dead girl lover who was really a sexually adventuresome older boy, there were hints of something that had yet to be told. There was body use and body pain; there was desire and betrayal and shame and compulsory concealment. Who inflicted these burns? After examining their position, I was sure they were not self-inflicted. I have never decoded his story. But of this I am sure: someone abused him, and that someone was both freed and implicated by his lies.

Bob made me think about the way tales of evil are told. Now I know that there are times when the fictive archives of narrative transformation can become history's most authentic messenger. By contrast, those "facts" that *can* be told seem flat and entombed, signifying nothing, as Bollas (1989) implies in his discussion of incest. For, as Pye (1996) suggests:

> The capacity to have memories at all, to have sufficient continuity of experience to have historicity, is dependent on our developing ability to engage in reverie and to imagine. . . . It is only as we come to be able to imagine, that we come to be able to remember" [p. 161].

To arrest the cycle of evil, we must know history. But in the reproductive cycle of evil, fact is always transmuted by lies, by the prohibition against telling, and by the imperative to tell. And even when traumatic memory can be told and is willing to be told, we must recall that trauma was not inscribed on a "blank slate." It was inscribed on the human unconscious. There, it was interwoven with developmental shifts in consciousness, cognition, affect, and perception, and with the dreamlike threads of human fantasy. And so, we cannot hope to encounter veridical traumatic facts void of all fiction. And we cannot allow fictive elements to void the very truths that fiction attempts to both convey and disguise. When our patient is suffering from a core of psychological deadness, there is a story among other stories that "cannot be told . . . the very act of telling (creating) a story is a lie, a charade. Paradoxically, the lie and the recognition of its falsehood in the context of an analytic discourse is the only locus of truth" (Ogden, 1997, pp. 68–69). The lie is the locus of the truth because "the fundamental problem the habitual liar is bringing to analysis by lying is primitive, and primarily involves not the truth and falsity of propositions *but the truth and falsity of his objects—their genuineness or deceitfulness*" (O'Shaughnessy, 1990, p. 187; italics added).

When we encounter a patient who is a liar, we must know he lies, and yet, we must know that the dead self was defined in *real* conditions of terror. We must not allow ourselves to be ensnared by the popular polarity of fact *or* fantasy. And we must not allow ourselves to be seduced into a purely narrative endeavor. In the context of evil, the analyst must recognize that imaginative narrative does not simply lead to imaginative narrative in infinite hermeneutic regress. Narrative is an elliptical and elusive pathway to the traumatic something *that really happened*. History vanishes and is transformed even as it is revealed. Imagination leads to facts, and facts to imagination.

Of all the facts that organize our daily existence, the fact of annihilation most compels us with its objective status precisely because it *is* a fact of annihilation. And yet, because this fact is a fact of annihilation, it seems to continually elude us. As analysts, we must aspire toward that element of historical truth that persists in the labyrinth of narration, even as absolute knowing often remains an impossibility. We must persist in attempts to know historical truth because it is the truth of oppression.

In a benign relationship of mutuality, one may safely relinquish rigid adherence to objective truth and mutually play with continually shifting realities. It is possible to find that space which Ogden (1997) calls the "intersubjective third": the mutual transformation of two equally legitimate perspectives on experience and reality. The relationship itself provides the ground that makes this transformation possible. But in the moment of annihilation there is no space for multiple perspective taking, for the containment of two subjectivities. Annihilation *is* the destruction of one subjectivity. Thus, the truth of annihilation is the harsh objective truth of domination. Powerless people can free themselves only by differentiating between actual truth and the lies that perpetuate the needs and objectives of their oppressor. Victims become powerful by repossessing the truth of their own condition. Anticipating this, the victimizer always engages in the falsification of history. Orwell (1949) captures this process when he writes of doublethink:

> The process has to be conscious or it would not be carried out with sufficient precision, but it also has to be unconscious or it would bring with it a feeling of falsity and hence of guilt. To tell deliberate lies while genuinely believing in them, to forget any fact that has become inconvenient and then, when it becomes necessary again, to draw it back from oblivion for just so long as it is needed, to deny the existence of objective reality and on the whole to take account of the reality which one denies—all this is indispensably necessary. Even in using the word doublethink it is necessary to exercise doublethink, for by using the word one admits that one is tampering with reality; by a fresh act of doublethink one erases this knowledge; and so on indefinitely with the lie always one leap ahead of the truth. Ultimately, it is by means of doublethink that the Party has been able to arrest the course of history [p. 36].

Tracing the history of destruction requires us to penetrate the reversals and inversions of doublethink. We are compelled to analyze fantasy in the pursuit of fact, and we are compelled to analyze fact in pursuit of fantasy, never forgetting that it is the *fact* of annihilation that has been the victim's oppressor. The difficulty of such a task must not cause our retreat. In our effort to repossess the marginalized truths of the oppressed (see Foucault, 1980), we must not remarginalize these truths in the bankruptcy of excessive relativism. We must not succumb to the erasure of a man's history, when that history has already been foreclosed by violence. Loftus (1991) resonates with this dilemma when she describes her deliberations about whether to testify against the Treblinka survivors who identified Ivan the Terrible. As a Jew, she cannot bear to engage in discrediting the memories of these survivors; she writes: "How can you separate a man from his memory? If you take the memories away, haven't you also stripped him of his past . . . without his memories, wouldn't [he] fold up and die, an exterior scaffolding that has lost its inner structure and suddenly collapses in upon itself?" (p. 231). We cannot deprive the survivor of his inner structure. We must draw ever closer to *what really happened*, and also to knowing that what really happened, happened in obscurity.

## BARBARA: INTIMATE BETRAYAL AND THE FORECLOSURE OF HISTORY

In the second year of her analysis, an intelligent, outspoken young woman tells me the following dream: "An envelope containing pornographic photographs and pamphlets about incest is delivered to my house. One of the pamphlets is about a seminar that has already passed; the second seminar is in October and has not yet been held. The girl in the pornographic photographs looks like me, at around the age of 11 or 12. I, too, had long hair at age 12. I am not sure what is happening in the picture. I think the girl is posing nude. There is writing next to the picture of the girl but I am not sure what it says. I was terrified." At this point, my patient begins sobbing and says, with fear and tentative conviction, "Did my father do this to me, take these pictures?"

Let us move back in time in her analysis, to the evolution of this moment. This woman entered treatment because of panic attacks and the disturbing memory of having been sexually abused by a female neighbor when she was five, a memory she never repressed. As we worked on this experience and began investigating the larger context of her life, we moved into a long period revealing profound anxiety and rage in relation to men. In addition to her panic attacks, she had night terrors and nightmares, extensive, shifting somatic complaints, rage storms at her otherwise beloved husband, and fears of rape and of looking womanly in front of men. She gained weight and began to dress so as to obscure her feminine beauty. She recalled a long period of engaging in degrading promiscuous sexuality at the behest of abusive boyfriends, and two date rapes. Her stepfather (the patient never knew her natural father; the mother married the stepfather when the patient was an infant) was initially presented as the preferred parent: intelligent, sophisticated, attentive, exciting, and interested in encouraging the patient in her explorations of life. She could confide in him and he in her. While the mother provided solid basic care, she was seen as cold and dull; it was clearly the stepfather who possessed the capacity to know her. She had not revealed the sexual abuse to either parent at the time it occurred, but, as an adult, she chose to tell her stepfather and not her mother.

Over time, another picture of her stepfather emerged: that of an alcoholic con man and pathological liar who had been arrested and jailed for embezzlement when she was three, after which the parents divorced. When she asked him why he was in jail, he lied to her, denying he had committed the thefts, although her mother unequivocally states he stole and conned over a long period of time. Throughout her adulthood, he presented himself as a retired attorney, who would sometimes take on clients. He talked about his law school days, his moneyed life as a successful attorney. And indeed she remembered his opulent homes, the trips to elegant restaurants. During treatment she found out that he had never been to law school, had taken no bar exam; his only proximity to law had been as a reasonably successful criminal.

My patient also revealed considerable material about her stepfather's sexual perversity, which involved orgies and compulsive affairs, which he told her about when she was a teenager; pornographic photos and letters about wife swapping; his insistence on kissing her on the mouth despite her obvious discomfort and attempts to evade him; the ways he related to her as his emotional wife instead of as his daughter; his efforts to take her with him to a nudist colony as a child despite her protests and humiliation; how even now he demands sexual admiration from her. When drunk at a recent party, he pulled her close and whispered seductively in her ear, "Give me a kiss." In the same period were a series of graphic sexual nightmares. She dreamt about huge penises bearing down on her face; about rape, vaginal pain and bleeding; about worms emerging from her vagina and rectum; about meeting the author of a book on incest and thanking her for writing a book "for me." In one image, she came to a party dressed in a short, tight sexy red dress (something she would never do) and was disturbed to encounter the teenage boy who had raped her. In the dream, this teenage rapist kissed her in exactly the way her stepfather does; she was mute and resistant in the same way she is with her stepfather. She has shared with me a growing suspicion that she was sexually abused by a man in her childhood, although she has no clear memories. When she talks about her suspicion, she is flooded by panic, but insists she wants to know if something happened. How can I know if he touched her? What I know is this: that she was both electrified and electrocuted by his oedipal seduction. She had surrendered to a man whose life was a construction of lies; she had believed his lies and known he was lying; she had coveted the truth and had eroticized the man he constructed with his illusions. And what I think is this: that a man driven by seduction and lies *could* molest his daughter; that a woman awakened and abandoned by the perversity of her stepfather could suspect that stepfather of incest when incest had not actually occurred.

On this particular day, she finally asked, "could my father have done this to me, taken these pictures?" I have just read yet another media exposé on the false memory controversy. I realize that this outspoken, serious, and assertive woman would confront her stepfather if thoroughly convinced that he had had incest with her. This litigious, volatile man would lie and very possibly sue me for "implanting" an incest memory. Her stepfather suddenly appears to me powerful, vindictive, and relentless in his retaliation; I am helpless, vulnerable, small. I feel exposed. There is a dangerous secret about what is going on in her analysis. I will be implicated. Financially ruined, professionally humiliated. I am a little girl, terrorized, with a shameful secret. Even as she weeps, she does not yet know, but she has lost me. I hear the voice of judicial accusation: Have I suggested these ideas? How can I demonstrate that I have not? Should I start taping sessions to protect myself, and how to explain this taping to the patient? Have I allowed her to be too literal in her interpretations of her dreams and symptoms? How can

I demonstrate in court that I have not led the patient into this accusation of incest?

Suddenly I feel I must demonstrate to the patient that these images may be more symbolic than literal, and possibly expressive of other dynamic issues. Because I am so anxious, I cannot sustain a therapeutic stance which apprehends the complex elaborations of fact and fantasy, memory and imagination. Regardless of whether she was the victim of actual incest, I know her to be trau-matized. And I know that to be traumatized is to be immersed in the contradictions of certainty and doubt. But I cannot locate our work between certainty and doubt. I want the definitiveness of documentation, notes in black and white, videotapes, evidence, the indisputable hard data of my therapeutic interventions. I must be able to show the courts that I explored other explanations besides incest for her dreams and symptoms. I must be able to show the stepfather that *I* do not accuse him. In the hardness of evidence I will leave her and find my own protection. Even as she weeps, I question her differently, drawing her away from the image of actual incest. Where I had been neutral in her quest, I am neutral no longer. She attempts to follow me where I am going, desperate for us to stay together, willing to be confused, deflected.

Do it to Julia. In this most critical moment of revelation, her trusted analyst-of-mutuality has been eclipsed first by a dissociated terrorized child, and then by the analyst-father-of-domination. I save myself by sacrificing my patient, my child, by repudiating her questions about her own history. I am inauthentic, subtly coercive and secretly ashamed. It is one of my worst moments as an analyst. I don't want her or anyone else to see me.

The next day I receive a rare call of protest from my patient; fortunately, I have been trustworthy up until now. By the time she calls, I have worked myself through this countertransferential moment. She says that she felt I did not believe her. She has never felt so alone and bewildered with me before. I know now that my failure is not a failure of belief. My failure is the refusal to remain in the dangerous place between certainty and doubt, memory and imagination. My failure is in the desire to construct a hard objec-tive history which occludes an emerging truth and sequesters me from danger. Despite my inquiry into how she perceived me in this therapeutic moment, she cannot allow herself to attribute her panic and confusion to any failure of mine, but rather must attribute this to her own lack of clarity and poor communication. This sophisticated woman, who is fully informed about the false-memory controversy and its attendant lawsuits etc., cannot access any of her knowledge about what may have actually occurred inside *me* during her session. This is familiar analytic ground for us: we have often seen a surge of panic attacks when she is refusing to know what she knows about being betrayed and in danger. In the transference, she resurrects an object tie of mendacity and submission, after I have enacted a subtle form of domination by redirecting the question of incest. She has returned to her bond with her stepfather, a bond in which all dangerous knowledge must be falsified and denied.

In subsequent sessions, she does not mention either incest or the moment of analytic rupture I have described. Her symptoms increase. She has retreated from what she was wondering about him, and what she knows about me, because I have reenacted the process of memory falsification. Her inability to know what she knows becomes the focus of her analysis. What she cannot yet afford to discover is that, unlike her father, I am willing to see myself and for her to see me, for her to see and know my betrayal, for her to be angry, for her to regain her memory and her history in this therapeutic moment. Now, together, we can newly define traumatic history as both interpretable and immutable, poised between certainty and doubt. And we will attempt to know what really happened with her stepfather, knowing that what really happened, happened in obscurity.

# CHAPTER 4

# THE PARADOX OF INNOCENCE:
# DISSOCIATIVE STATES IN
# PERPETRATORS OF BODILY VIOLATION

❧

HE WAS ONE OF MY FIRST PATIENTS; one of several perpetrators whose treatment narrative would form a dissociative confession of crimes known and yet not known. Prior to his retirement, David had been a night healthcare worker caring for the aged and terminally ill in a chaotic, deteriorated city hospital. By day David would become inert, retreating to a dirty bed in a cramped city apartment. Like a mole in the dark of night, he would emerge to maintain disintegrated bodies as they lay dying. Rarely engaging with others, David's human contact was restricted to the bodies of his patients and the bodies he encountered in orgies. Too old now to be desirable for anonymous sex, and retired from his hospital position, the loss of skin-to-skin contact left him anxious and desolate. He now lived exclusively within the deep schizoid silence of his dismal retreat, wrapped in a somnolent cocoon. Complaining for the first time of what he called "loneliness" and depression, he sought treatment in a mental health clinic. His family history was sparsely and numbly provided but was remarkable for its physical abuse and extreme emotional barrenness. Through a dissociative maze of communication the patient revealed the fact that he had committed multiple acts of sex abuse and murder with his needy patients. Gradually, a picture emerged of a man who exposed himself to patients and masturbated them, and who also selectively "euthanized" them by refusing to provide the emergency medical care they begged from him. He experienced himself as responding to their wordless needs to be soothed and helped to die (despite their manifest demands for continued medical intervention). Even as I pursued supervisory, legal, and ethical advice, the patient steadfastly maintained a profound experience of himself as decent and blandly innocent. Any attempt to translate his euphemistic statements, insinuations, and paranoid reversals into language like "exposing himself," "sexual molestation," or "killing" was met with outraged innocence and elaborate rationalizations. Extensive inquiry indicated that he had only committed these acts with his patients, and that he had no intention of seeking new objects for "acts of mercy." My counsel did not consider him to be currently dangerous; I was required to maintain confidentiality about past crimes and continue the treatment. Ultimately, the patient "terminated" me in response to my efforts to examine his splitting, denial, and dissociation. Emerging with his life-lie intact, *this lonely and decent man* returned to the coffin of his existence and closed its lid. He left within me the horror and inarticulate memory of sex abuse and murder.

Many years later, a middle-class attorney was convicted of battering his child to death. The evidence was certain, the conviction swift and ready. And yet, he gave a remarkable and haunting television interview. His face haggard with grief and bewildered persecution, he wept compelling tears for the loss of his child. He protested that he missed his daughter and that he had not killed her. His version of events was vastly at odds with the one that emerged at his trial. This image resonated with my experience with patients like David. I recall thinking that this father was not simply lying; *he was telling the truth*. How was his internal world constructed so that he was able to experience himself as innocent?

The thrust of this chapter is to penetrate the internal dissociative state of the perpetrator: a state of felt innocence in a condition of actual guilt. Although the frequent denials and cognitive distortions of pedophiles have been well documented (Abel et al., 1989; Hayashino, Wurtele, and Klebe, 1995), contemporary investigations into the fallibility of memory focus exclusively on the survivor (Brenneis, 1994; Lindsay and Read, 1994; Lynn and Nash, 1994) and lack a depth analysis of the perpetrator. Here I will initiate such an analysis by examining a particular type of perpetrator: one who is himself or herself a survivor of incest or child abuse (Groth, 1982). Unlike the knowing psychopath, whose menacing lies and mystifications are intended to retain power and dominance, this type of perpetrator is profoundly schizoid. He or she possesses an incestuous self that *lives without speech, without consciousness, and without memory.* This perpetrator–survivor has entered the "black hole" of nameless dread, in which hope has been surrendered, integrity has been foreclosed, and the soul is forfeit (Grotstein, 1990). He is a schizoid who engages in evil without love or hate, but rather to control emergent internal states that he fears but never enters. His abusive self exists in a kind of remoteness, deeply sequestered from other, more accessible selves. He experiences neither the sense of being really real in relation to the outside world (Bromberg, 1984), nor of any true internal values or deep emotion (Meltzer, 1975). Shengold (1989) comments that a "hypnotic living deadness, a state of existing 'as if' one were there, is often the result of chronic early overstimulation or deprivation. . . . But the automaton has murder within him" (p. 25). In Sartre's (1956) terms, this is a perpetrator who cannot recognize the subjectivity of the other without becoming an "it" in someone else's universe. In order for him to become fully human he must, like Camus's (1956) judge/penitent, turn inward on himself, becoming truly alive only at the very moment when he is absolutely known and absolutely condemned. Only with the recognition of his own guilt can the victimized child within him emerge as authentically innocent at last. This is a terrifying journey into emotional terrors and social repudiation; how many possess such a longing to become human and such moral courage?

As I focus on the perpetrator here, I must emphasize my broader framework, which places incest in a dyadic system of mutual dissociation. This system involves shifting intersubjective states that render problematic the mutual *simultaneous* recovery and recognition of the historical facts of sexual abuse. These shared states of mutual dissociation are viewed as an elaborate, cocon-structed intersubjective universe, the very amniotic fluid in which the perpetrator-survivor relationship develops and assumes its shape. The perpetrator lives in possession of the victim's innocence while the victim lives in possession of the perpetrator's guilt. For the mutual *simultaneous* recognition of incest to occur, both must awaken at once to their actual condition: one innocent and one guilty. Without doubt, it is in the perpetrator's interest to retain the dark power of his lies. However, I will speculate that, within his own depersonalized and derealized state, the perpetrator-survivor can also genuinely experience himself as innocent, or experience his or her acts as not really *real*, not really *abuse*, or perhaps, not really *his*. Further, I would argue that a perpetrator's awakened depressive capacity for reparation and remorse is cocreated by the survivor's rage and recovery of memory, while the survivor's recov-ery of rage and memory awaits the perpetrator's recognition (Grand, 1995) (see also Conclusion in chapter 8). Thus the emer-gence of delayed memories of incest (for both perpetrator and sur-vivor) seems caught in an eternal intersubjective loop, in which each seeks the prior recognition of the subjective other to relin-quish the mutual sleep of not-knowing. One can imagine the rar-ity with which this cataclysmic shift actually occurs between perpetrator and victim; thus mutual simultaneous linguistically shared historical knowing between perpetrator and survivor becomes virtually impossible. Generally the survivor's ability to know evolves through engaging this intersubjective shift in the analysis, through the empathic recognition of the perpetrator-within-the analyst (Grand, 1995). It is often the case that this occurs only after the perpetrator dies or is otherwise disempow-ered (Lionells, 1995, personal communication). The perpetrator's capacity to know his own incestuous acts may be likewise awak-ened through an encounter with the "objective hatred" of a vic-tim surrogate within the analyst or society.

In this chapter, perpetrators' illusions of innocence are investi-gated within the context of two contemporary theoretical trends: the new relational view of self as multiple (Bromberg, 1993; Mitchell, 1993a,b), and the reformulation of Kleinian theory proposed by Mitrani (1994a,b) and Ogden (1989). Both formulations share remarkable resonance with the view of memory and dissociation emerging from trauma theory and research. They provide a psychoanalytic level of understanding for such phenomena as: derealization and disembodiment; loss of agency; altered and coconscious states; the prelinguistic, somatic encoding of traumatic memory; and the severing of connections between events and their affects and meanings (Krystal, 1988; Putnam, 1990; Herman, 1992; Reis, 1993; Davies and Frawley, 1994; Van der Kolk, 1996). These dissociative sequelae of incest inform what I call "traumatically induced disorders of knowing" (Grand, 1995; see also Kramer, 1983; Laub and Auerhahn, 1993; Price, 1995).

A synthesis of empirical and psychoanalytic perspectives on disorders of knowing allows for a beginning phenomenology of felt innocence in a condition of actual guilt. Such a phenomenology must be embedded in the newly emergent view of traumatic memory and self organization, a view that emphasizes fragmentation, dissociation, and the lack of linear, symbolic encoding. I particularly agree with Reis (1995) that Ogden's (1989) reformulation of Kleinian theory has comprehensive implications for the understanding of the survivor–perpetrator's conviction of innocence. Here, I briefly elucidate the relevant premises of Ogden's theory. I then move to focus more narrowly on what Mitrani (1994a,b) calls the adhesive pseudo-object relatedness.

## THE MULTIPLICITY OF SELVES-IN-RELATION AND THE DESTRUCTION OF LINKAGES

Mitchell (1993a,b), and Bromberg (1993) have reframed our theories of self and unconscious in a manner that permits us to begin integrating psychoanalytic theories of schizoid phenomena with the trauma literature on dissociation. The dynamics of delayed memory as well as the phenomenology of felt innocence in conditions of actual guilt become comprehensible with this new look at the self.

According to Mitchell, the self does not begin as a unitary phenomenon that then fragments under the cumulative weight of conflictual object relations. His view of self involves a multiplicity of selves developed in a complex relational field. Health involves a relatively fluid access to these selves, and a general sense of comfortable containment of them. Illness in the multiplicity model may take either the form of an overly rigid, narrow, and inauthentic "life-lie" about the unitary nature of one's self or, with sufficient trauma, it may take the form of an agonizing incoherent array of disorganized and discontinuous self states (Harris, 1994). Within this conceptualization, unconscious contents are not repressed feelings and memories per se, but the *very selves* who have had these experiences (Bromberg, 1993). Mitchell (1993a,b) views the state of unconsciousness as characterized by the destruction of linkages between various self states. Previously, the unconscious was a spatial metaphor, a receptacle holding once-known conflictual material out-of-awareness. In this contemporary perspective, the unconscious now becomes a fluid temporal medium of not-knowing, of never-been-known, of not being real. Thus, whole selves disappear from "consciousness" and are like ghosts on a stage, enacting their presence, hoping to be heard and to be *not-heard*.

Searles (1959) offers an excellent clinical vignette that precisely illustrates this destruction of linkages. He describes a session with a female schizophrenic patient who, while passionately engaging him in an intense and provocative discussion of politics, simultaneously behaves in an extremely seductive manner. The linkage to her avowed, conscious self is missing. Searles experienced himself as prohibited from *knowing* the sexual relatedness; he was permitted only to engage with the political discussion. This conflict left him suffering from a welter of contradictory, not-to-be-known feelings and fantasies that resulted in a sense of being made crazy. Here, the heuristic value of the new view of the self is evident. Her sexual "self" was not-known; it was enacted and dissociated in much the way Bromberg describes. Whereas the unitary model would have been strained to account for such clinical phenomena, the new model readily accommodates the intersubjective states of dissociation characteristic of such patient–therapist, parent–child dyads.

Once we are able to view the personality as a system of selves-in-relation, and we understand unconsciousness and pathology to be defined by the relative lack of intactness of self-state linkages, we have the analytic concepts with which to enter the realm of incest, dissociation, and delayed memory. Intrinsic to the destruction of linkages is the loss of the memories belonging to the self who has lived them. Psychoanalytic theories of the traumatized schizoid self are at last emergent in the work of Davies and Frawley (1994). These authors have formulated descriptions of the dissociated internal object world of the incest survivor. Their perspective in conjunction with that of Alpert (1994) and others allows us to explicate the dynamics of delayed traumatic memory within a psychoanalytic framework. Such dynamics are applicable to perpetrator and survivor alike.

Inherent in the destruction of linkages between self states is the loss of the sense of agency, and of the embodied self. These two essential deficits characteristic of dissociation have been extensively described in the trauma literature (Ferenczi 1932; Ehrenberg, 1987; Shengold, 1989; Putnam, 1990; Herman, 1992; Waites, 1993). As Mitchell (1993a) says, the recovery of a healthy capacity to contain a multiplicity of selves involves an increase in the sense of agency for one's actions and enactments; a recognition that what one does, one is. The lack of such containment results in a felt experience of passivity, of not being the agent of one's life, one's acts. One acts from one's body: to own one's acts, to be present in one's sensations and one's acts, is to be *embodied*.

Nowhere are the intersecting phenomena of dissociative selves, disembodiment, and loss of agency more vividly evoked than in the early work of R. D. Laing (1960), despite his somewhat outmoded adherence to a unitary model of self. For Laing, an onslaught of ontological terror results in the splitting of self into true and false selves; authentic experience is hidden from the external world and radically disembodied. The false self *becomes* the body; therefore, none of the actions and sensations of the body are experienced as really *real* or really *his*. Only the disembodied thoughts of the true self are real. The true self is experienced as profoundly honest and utterly divorced from the actions of the false self. Because any act is public and revealed, the true self has a terror of owning the act; to reveal itself in an act is to risk annihilation. As Laing (1960) says,

"There is something final and definitive about an act. . . . Action is the dead end of possibility. . . . If it cannot be eschewed, then every act must be of such an equivocal nature that the self can never be trapped in it" (p. 8). Laing describes a schizoid patient who, discussing his biweekly sex life with his wife, says he never *really* had sex with his wife. According to Laing, if the patient were psychotic (or more severely dissociated) he would say, instead, he *never* had sex with his wife, that *he* never had sex with his wife, or that she is not *his* wife. The true self experiences no contradiction in its disavowal of the body's actions and its simultaneous conviction of radical honesty. *The true self is experienced as authentically innocent of the actions of the body.*

Thus, even Hamlet, one of literature's greatest opponents of evil and its mendacity, can disavow responsibility for the murder of Laertes's father:

> What I have done
> That might your nature, honor, and exception
> Roughly awake, I here proclaim was madness.
> Was't Hamlet wronged Laertes? Never Hamlet.
> If Hamlet from himself be ta-en away,
> And when he's not himself does wrong Laertes,
> Then Hamlet does it not, Hamlet denies it.
> Who does it then? His madness. If't be so,
> Hamlet is of the faction that is wronged;
> His madness is poor Hamlet's enemy.
> Sir, in this audience,
> Let my disclaiming from a purposed evil
> Free me so far in your most generous thoughts
> [*Hamlet,* act 5, scene 2].

Madness has divorced Hamlet from his body, and so he can protest innocence of a murder which has been committed by his own hand.

Whether the act is experienced as an event happening *to* a passive self, or as something initiated by a self who is not-me, the end result is the same: a subjective experience of the act as not really *real* and not really *mine*. We begin to see how one might authentically experience oneself as innocent of acts committed by dissociated selves. It is noteworthy that clinical examples of disembodiment and loss of agency frequently involve disavowed sexual activity. Perhaps the intense sensory/affective experience of sexuality, with its attendant altered states, makes it particularly prone to autistic usage of the other and the destruction of linkages. Certainly, the actions and sensations of the body are a primary theater for the enactments of ghost selves; a theater where they may speak without being known. As Laing (1960) writes (quoting Hegel): "The act is 'simple, determinate, universal.' But his self wishes to be complex, indeterminate, unique. The act is 'what can be said of it.' But he must never be what can be said of him. He must remain ungraspable, elusive, transcendent" (pp. 87–88).

## THE EMBEDDEDNESS OF HISTORY, EVIL, AND DISSOCIATION: A NEO-KLEINIAN PERSPECTIVE

The multiplicity of selves and the destruction of linkages provides us with a beginning phenomenology of the conviction of innocence in a condition of actual guilt. This phenomenology will be considerably enriched by a neo-Kleinian understanding of developmental modalities. In essence, I propose that trauma induces death anxiety; this death anxiety is metabolized and redissociated through pathological, narcissistic modalities. When massive trauma occurs in childhood, mature empathic modes of being may never have been consolidated, and the personality is perennially rooted in narcissistic terrors and narcissistic forms of defense (Balint, 1968; Stolorow and Lachmann, 1980; Little, 1985). In a sense, my perspective integrates existentialist and neo-Kleinian theories. Existentialism focuses on the dread of death, on the loneliness and freedom that dread can inspire, as well as on the destructive characterological self-deceptions through which we take flight from that dread (Laing, 1960; Becker, 1973; 1975; Yalom, 1980; May, 1981; etc.). Neo-Kleinian theory (e.g., Riviere, 1964; Grotstein,

1979; Klein, 1983; Ogden, 1989) provides a language for the demonic pursuits through which mankind takes flight from his dread, as well as a developmental map of death anxiety.

Like Alford (1997), I suggest that pathological forms of developmental modalities potentiate specific malevolent defenses against annihilation anxiety. But I propose something more: that malignant dissociative contagion finds its roots in both the autistic–contiguous and paranoid–schizoid modalities, because each mode not only potentiates the destructive use of the other, it also *disrupts the capacity for historical memory and personal accountability*. Neo-Kleinian theory implicitly articulates the mutual embeddedness of history, evil, and dissociation; it is therefore unique in its capacity to penetrate the paradox of innocence in the survivor-perpetrator. While this chapter focuses on the adhesive modality, chapters 5 and 6 are devoted to other developmental modes and to their unique impact on malignant dissociative contagion.

Unlike Klein's unitary, sequential model of the paranoid-schizoid and depressive positions, Ogden's (1989) reformulation of these positions as dialectically coexistent *modes* of experience resonates with the new view of self as multiple. Health and pathology are similarly defined: health involves the fluid adaptive accessibility of different modalities (Ogden, 1989); pathology is characterized by the inaccessibility of a particular modality (Ogden, 1989), and by various degrees of dissociative discontinuities of self (Grotstein, 1981). In illness, shifting coexistent self states, each characterized by its own anxiety, are *unknown to one another*. Dissociative shifts occur between narcissistic and object relatedness; between symbolic speech and the archaic viscera; between the struggle over being and the surrender to mourning; between destruction and empathy. Finally, and most important, these dissociative shifts move between modalities characterized by continuous memory, and those that are ahistorical. These discontinuous states often exist without memory, primarily because both the autistic–contiguous and paranoid–schizoid modes are intrinsically *ahistorical*; it is only in the depressive mode that historicity is created and a continuous autobiographical self exists (Ogden, 1989). Acts committed outside the depressive mode may be said to exist outside of self-reflexive, discursive memory; they are neither forgotten nor repressed. In the autistic–contiguous mode, experience is sensory, prelinguistic, and devoid of agency. As I describe in greater depth below, acts committed in this modality exist only in the ephemeral somatic present and never become linguistically encoded. In the paranoid–schizoid mode, splitting and projective identification function to *disappear* goodness from badness. The incapacity for ambivalence continually gives rise to *new, ahistorical* images of self and other as purely loving or hating; memory and continuity is foreclosed. Instead of historicity there is "a continual defensive recasting of the past" (Ogden, 1989, p. 13). For Ogden, both autistic–contiguous and paranoid–schizoid modes lack an interpreting subject who can *know his own history, and know himself as agent.* This incapacity to know oneself as historical agent is exacerbated by paranoid–schizoid attacks on linkages (Grotstein, 1981). The destruction of linkages *is* the destruction of thought and perception; experience is rendered insignificant and meaningless, and "the significance of *facts for truth* undergoes eclipse or extinction" (Grotstein, 1981, p. 93). This recognition of discontinuous ahistorical states and modalities is embedded in Klein's appreciation of human malignancy and destruction. Such a model provides a map of human darkness, readily locating the shifts and contradictions in the perpetrator's authentic levels of destruction and empathy, object relatedness and narcissistic usage, memory and oblivion.

It is only within the depressive mode that an interpreting subject emerges who knows history as continuous: as both interpretable and *nonetheless immutable* (Ogden, 1989). This capacity is simultaneous to the emergence of object relatedness, empathy, guilt, remorse, and the capacity for agency. For my present purposes it is critical to note that the birth of a historical subject is simultaneous to the birth of authentic object-related empathy and concern. Although various types of love and passion derive from the autistic–contiguous and paranoid–schizoid modes, they are, in themselves, more prone to the narcissistic usage of the other. Thus, the *lack* of a historical subject is inherently associated with those modalities in which the other may be used either in the pursuit of autistic–contiguous sensory exploitation *or* in the service of the splitting and projective identification of hatred and destruction. Where linkages to the depressive mode have collapsed, and annihilation anxiety is prevalent, where the interpersonal environment of trauma has potentiated the renewal of cruelty, trauma is readily transmuted into acts of evil, and the perpetrator identifies with the aggressor (A. Freud, 1966). In modalities void of agency and of history, various types and degrees of felt innocence are inevitable.


## THE VIOLATING "ADHESIVE" SELF AND ITS DISINTEGRATIVE ANXIETIES

In this chapter, my focus is on primitive states of somatic disintegration, states in which evil may be perpetrated without history or desire. Ogden's (1989) autistic–contiguous mode of experience, and Mitrani's (1994a,b) concept of "adhesive pseudo-object relations" provide an excellent framework for this investigation.

Ogden, Mitrani, and others (Bick, 1968; Meltzer, 1975) have articulated a sensory, presymbolic narcissistic modality that precedes (and subsequently coexists with) Klein's paranoid–schizoid and depressive modes. This "autistic contiguous" or "adhesive" mode focuses on the creation of a psychic skin that functions as an ontological container for fragmentary chaotic bits of mind. The intactness of psychic skin allows for a sense of continuous and coherent existence. This skin barrier generates a rudimentary distinction between inside and outside, self and other, and gives rise to the phenomena of felt agency. According to Ogden (1989), psychic skin derives from, and is sustained by, the continuous benign rhythms and textures of environmental sensation. Elsewhere, Grand and Alpert (1993) have argued that the inescapable impingement of incest shatters the child's experience of benign sensory contiguities, destroying the containing psychic skin. Existential terrors precipitate a search for the restoration of being through the establishment of sensory containment. Thus, incest gives birth to an "adhesive" self. This self does not experience itself as acting on the world, but rather as a mass of chaotic bits that either does or does not have being and a containing membrane. This self is lived in the body and *not-known*. There is no mentation from which to initiate an act and no linguistic symbolization with which to encode it in memory.

This self is characterized by what Mitrani (1994a) calls "adhesive pseudo-object relations" in which others function as utilitarian sources of sensory contiguities, and are experienced as insensate, inanimate, and without interior (also Krystal, 1988). Because the adhesive self has not entered the paranoid–schizoid or depressive modes, there is no sense of love or hate, of goodness or badness, of guilt or remorse in the adhesive use of the other; there is only sensation. Such "adhesive" usage can involve ordinary forms of narcissistic relatedness. However, it is significant that Mitrani's (1994b) clinical example of such pseudo-object relations is that of a fictional serial killer. Similarly, I suggest that the adhesive use of the other can include abusive sexual contacts. Where Mitrani is not concerned with questions of memory and history, I will argue that the presymbolic nature of the adhesive self intrinsically produces sensory exploitations that are not encoded in discursive memory as *acts on someone else's body*. For such a perpetrator, there is no living interior to the surface body he adheres to while creating his second skin. Not an agent, but rather a trope, he lives in diffuse, prelinguistic sensory and affective states, shifting in the direction of an enlivening sensory medium with which to ease the terror of the "black hole." *The innocence of traumatized childhood and the guilt of incestuous perpetration are thus located and confounded in the same sequestered wordless self.*[1] At the same time, this primitive, prelinguistic adhesive self may exist on a dual or multiple track with other selves and modalities characterized by more sophisticated levels of relatedness and symbolization (Ogden, 1989; Mitrani, 1994a,b). The incestuous self may be embedded in authentically alive, more object-related selves *whose linkages to the adhesive self are partially or completely lacking.* The malignant adhesive self may be

---

1. This view offers a psychoanalytic level of analysis for research findings that indicate the existence of a nonverbal, unsymbolized, visceral memory modality (Bucci, 1994) in which memory of trauma is deposited and from which it is reenacted outside of linguistic awareness (Van der Kolk, 1996).

encapsulated, presiding over a small but deadly zone in the self system. And it may move in and out of more empathic modes of being that do possess history and agency. The perpetrator may therefore demonstrate extraordinary shifts between goodness and badness. As Goldberg (1987) might suggest, such a perpetrator may distract herself from dissociative shifting so that she experiences and presents a "pseudo-integrated" mental state. Through these shifts, and through the seamless concealment of these shifts, the perpetrator engenders great confusion and paralysis in those around her.

The perpetrator's labyrinthine intersubjective operations about incestuous history become comprehensible if we contextualize the concept of the multiplicity of selves within the neo-Kleinian metaphor. While the adhesive self might commit incest without memory, intentionality, or desire, the paranoid-schizoid self might participate in sexual abuse in a more linguistically encoded, object-related and sadistic manner. This paranoid-schizoid self is more likely to be the self who knows and lies, demanding and perpetuating the master–slave relation (see chapters 5 and 6). If there is a depressive self, paranoid-schizoid memories may coexist with depression, remorse, and guilt. The perpetrator's personality resembles a Russian puzzle box, revealing separate, ever smaller, and seemingly infinite containers. This phenomenon begins to account for the often described experience of survivors that father raped them in the nighttime and seemed perfectly normal in the morning.

## DISSOCIATIVE CONFESSION AND THE ADHESIVE SELF

When the patient's "crime" is dissociatively communicated by disavowed selves, the analytic field becomes densely problematic. The analyst enters the same dissociative process that the perpetrator shared with his victim: was a *crime really committed*? If the "confession" involves the abuse of children, how do we assess the realities of abuse and the consequent necessity of reporting? The twin influences of the patient's denial and our own dawning horror may seduce us into not inquiring and not knowing, particularly when the perpetrator possesses a generally sophisticated, related, and likable self system. When the analyst does inquire and attempts to determine risk factors for continued abuse, another conundrum arises. What self is engaged with our inquiry and does it have linkages to the incestuous self? Can a speaking self know and give us assurances on behalf of a wordless, presymbolic, adhesive self?

Thus, legal and ethical concerns are embedded in a complex analytic process that partakes of the perpetrator's dissociative field. Future study of the analytic treatment of pedophiles must explore management issues and the clinical implications of reporting one's patient for sexual abuse. Such an investigation is beyond the scope of this chapter. In the cases presented here, reporting and case management were neither required nor appropriate. Where children were involved, the children are now adults. I have specifically selected these cases to minimize distraction from my central focus: that is, the adhesive nature of incest, and the patient's experience of the incestuous act as not really *real*, not really *mine*, or not really *sex*.

We now have the theoretical framework with which to understand the acute adhesive anxieties aroused in David during his work at the hospital. Daily, he had visual and tactile encounters with the sensory disintegration of his patients as they lay dying. It was as if he must continually witness the dissolution of intact skin membranes; as if he must watch his own dread awaken as minds fell through the holes in decaying skin surface. Lacking in any capacity to differentiate their bodies from his own, lacking in any mode of symbolic defense or containment, he must end this terrifying descent into bodiless fragmentation. And so, he engages in unsymbolized acts of sex abuse and murder. By masturbating them, he attempts to restore bodily sensation and cohesion. By killing them, he limits the spreading holes in the bodily container. He seals their holes and liberates himself from escalating fragmentation. For David, the primitive, dissociative process of the adhesive mode predominated a generally regressed self system, precluding any possible emergence of discursive knowing and depressive remorse.

In the following case vignette the patient is more genuinely engaged in treatment and the adhesive self is embedded in a more sophisticated, object-related self system. Linkages to symbolic self states are not entirely destroyed, allowing for various types and degrees of knowing and not knowing in the patient. With such patients, the analyst is placed in a paradoxical position: the capacity to know is at once more accessible and more remote. Where David was evidently bizarre and fit the expected image of a perpetrator, Michael possessed a respectable, high-functioning self system that made it difficult to recognize him as a perpetrator of incest.

Michael entered treatment because of marital discord. A successful retired businessman, his role in his family life is one of quiet disengagement; he is continually withdrawing from an angry, impassioned wife who rages at his disavowed provocations. He is intelligent, thoughtful, and slow-speaking; he is kind from a point of great remoteness. Each time he speaks he seems to be drawing together distant, alienated strands of experience from an inner well. The very act of self-reflective speech appears to entail an extraordinarily difficult process of *directing an inner search*. It is as if he is mentally translating from his speech into mine, as if speech itself is rooted in quicksand. As he struggles to articulate himself in emotional language, it becomes apparent that Michael has never experienced himself as an emotional agent in any of his life's events.

Blandly, he describes his neglectful, sexually demanding, and exhibitionistic mother; like his father, the patient met his mother's emotional and sexual onslaughts with stolid passivity. As he tells me, his speech is flat and his body is living. His voice is a hum, his words a dull link in a halting chain. At any time of day—morning, afternoon, evening—he renders me somnolent. His adhesive self announces its presence through the hum, through continual rubbing of various parts of his clothing, his hair, his skin. I feel his voice rubbing me, rubbing me, a masseur luring me into a disturbing sleep.

Sometimes he stutters, and the rubbing stutters and stops. I feel resentful, ruptured in soothing, jarred into wakefulness, but also ashamed of my sleepiness. I glance at his face, and he seems disorganized by pain. I ask him to tell me about his body, and he says he is cold and numb. His body is generally cold and numb *or* warm and numb. But sometimes, it is not numb. Now he associates to lifelong incidents of nameless dread and panic. What he fears he does not know. It is like a hovering thing that gnaws until it feels like a scream. He mentions the rough fabric on his chair and the itching sensations it generates. He begins to scratch, and he cannot stop scratching. His skin has always been sensitive. He cannot wear wool. There is another chair, covered with chintz: its surface is smooth, it has no texture, no stiff nub to invade him. But he cannot ask if he can move to the other chair. Session after session is interrupted by scratching, until I can no longer bear it and suggest he use the other chair. Now he resumes rubbing: rubbing the chintz, rubbing his arms, his clothing, his hair. It is more quiet than the scratching, less maddening to my body. It is like an arrest of the stuttering; in this quiescence, our bodies sigh with relief. Everything softens and goes quiet once again.

He had seemed intensely anxious as he described his physical discomforts. Now he seems intensely soothed. I inquire about the rubbing. At first he is surprised and says *he doesn't know he is doing it*; later he says he thinks he has been doing this since he was a child *although he never knew it*. He doesn't know what it means. One day, a blush emerges across his face and suffuses his entire body; he describes prickling hot sensations like needles penetrating his skin. He examines his arms to see if there is an outbreak of hives, and wonders if he is also allergic to the chintz. Now, there is nowhere left to go: wool or chintz, one chair or the other, his body cannot tolerate any placement or position. He describes a history of hives beginning in his late adolescence. I find myself mirroring his scratching, maddened with an itch, wishing I could remove my skin, scrub it down, replace it.

In the subsequent session, he haltingly reports having had an incestuous relationship with his younger sister. It seems she has now repudiated and condemned him for repeatedly sexually abusing her when she was 11 and he was 17. It suddenly becomes apparent that her rage was the true precipitant for his entering analysis. His wife's rage seems like an analogue for his sister's. His wife's anger is easier to speak of, and suffering it seems to have penitential significance for this man who has never made amends to his sister. His sister is not speaking to him, although she has spoken to his wife. They seem to sympathize with one another about Michael's emotional unresponsiveness, about his provocative disavowals of responsibility. His wife considers divorce. Both women are united in the desire to sever all connection with him. Dimly, he fears their abandonment, but cannot act to prevent it, much as he could not switch chairs.

In speaking of incestuous memory, Michael has always remembered the *fact* of the sexuality, but he is injured by his sister's perception of him as an *abuser*. He feels unjustly accused and persecuted by a histrionic sister; believing she is manipulated by 12-step groups and therapists into seeing herself as a victim. He recalls the sexuality between them as pleasant and consensual if embarrassing. While he acknowledges that it was *really incest*, it was not *really* traumatic, nor was it really *he* who perpetrated it. Although he is able to report that he initiated the sex, he was not *really the agent of it; he was not really six years older, physically larger and more powerful, and in a superior familial power position, and she was not really a child.* And while he dimly acknowledges some marital difficulties, he feels unjustly persecuted by his wife's accusations, and feels victimized by her threats of divorce. He is a good man, a good provider, loyal, reliable. Her complaints are insubstantial, her vision of "intimacy" overly romantic, her emotions dramatic.

As a professional, as an athlete, he has led a life of agentic success. As a neighbor, and as a friend, he is perceived as kind, helpful, generous, a "brick" in times of trouble. He has been welcomed, invited, celebrated, enjoyed. But with women, there is a collapse of all sense of emotional agency; with them, Michael cannot imagine having impact on another. In the dimming of all emotion, he also cannot imagine another having impact upon him. He cannot visualize human relations as a mutual, living system of engagement and accountability. It is apparent that he has neither experienced his own anguish in relation to his mother nor his own culpability in relation to his sister. He is an isolate. Emotional input and output are barred from experience, hidden within his sensory anxieties and his gestures toward adhesive containment.

In the session after the incest revelation, we focus more on the sensory anxieties evoked, for example, by the chair fabrics. We move back and forth between body states and body memories, inquiring into the beginnings of his hives, his itch, his rubbing. For me, it is apparent that the fabric *is* the everpresent maternal body. He is flooded by the sense of being intolerably invaded and over-stimulated by his mother's sexual touch and exhibitionism. He had no escape: it was coming in at his eyes, at his skin; through all his senses, with the scent of her perfume, and the filmy presence of erotic negligees. Through my own body somnolence, he evokes the cloying silks, the cool satins flowing along her body, flowing from her body to his limbs, luring him into a disturbing surren-der. He can remember a steamy bathroom filled with oils and foaming salts. He can remember his mother asking him to bring her a drink as she languished in her bath, her breasts barely con-cealed beneath the opulent surface of bubbles and water.

And then he can remember her looking at his erect penis and laughing. Laughing because he is small, and erect and desirous, laughing because she is sexual and alluring and more potent than his small powers. He recalls overhearing her tell her friend that she was "concerned" that he was "small." His shame was deep, and his rage was annihilating. If she didn't want him, why did she invite him? If he was a child, why did she seduce him? He can remem-ber her dancing with other men, and laughing later about their passes: fat fools, bald men, what were they thinking? She was the uncontested femme fatale of all social occasions, sometimes sleep-ing with other men, sometimes not. Flowers were delivered, letters received, accepted, refused. Days were spent shopping, manicuring, exercising, languishing by the pool, receiving massage. Parental functions were provided by a series of matronly housekeepers. Dinner was served, not made. Offhanded, she would run her fin-gers through his hair and ask if he was a good boy, was his home-work done? And he remembers a few abortive assertions by his father, accusations that she was flirting. His mother ridiculed his father as she had ridiculed Michael in the bathroom, deriding his manliness, saying he was lucky to keep her, that he was only good for making money. And his father took it. Adoring, denying her adultery, he was grateful for her small attentions, for her presence on his arm.

Remembering the scene in the bathroom, it was as if Michael's entire skin surface were penetrated by hot needles. He feels his viscera coming apart and disintegrating. At such moments his rubbing of his skin, hair, and clothes intensifies; he seeks a soothing restitution of his bodily integrity. At home, he masturbates compulsively, seeking his intact penis, seeking sensation. He comes to realize that his sister's young body served the same function: her skin on his skin felt soothing, quieting; utterly unlike the intense violation of his mother's touch. And if he was "small," she was smaller; his penis filled her holes. Slowly, through our movement in and out of memory and body sensation, a new empathic remorse awakened in him about violating his sister. His adhesive self formed links to his depressive self. He had always possessed a "depressive self" living in relation to work, neighbors, friends. But this depressive self had rarely existed in his transactions with his sister and his wife. Now his adhesive and depressive selves join in his memory of incest and in his understanding of his marriage. He understood his sexual violation of his sister as both tragic and inevitable. Now he remembers his sister's body as it was, a child's body, untouched and inviolate. He realizes that his sister was a *child* and that she experienced his touch as he experienced his mother's: violating, humiliating, and disintegrative. Now, he realizes his own schizoid insularity, his passivity, and begins to comprehend his wife's frustrations. A sense of agency is born within him as he simultaneously recognizes himself both as an *innocent* child victim and as a *guilty* incestuous perpetrator. Slowly, he embarks on the path of emotional restitution, with his wife, with his sister, with himself.

I have worked with perpetrators who possess relatively intact linkages and some depressive capacity for remorse. Even they have difficulty fully recovering memory and emerging from dissociative splits. A frequent condition for the recovery of this type of perpetrator's memory is an encounter with the "objective hatred" (Winnicott, 1958) of their victim, the analyst or society. Such hatred may function to allow the survivor-perpetrator to locate his own rage and childhood victimization at last. In so doing, he may emerge from his own dissociative haze and begin to forge an identification with his own victimized child, rather than with his own perpetrator parent. As Frederickson (1990) suggests, the only empathic position to offer the abuser is a position that allows the abusing self to finally enter its own affective states rather than to flee the "black hole" and continue parental reenactments. In Mitchell's (1993a) terms, the encounter with objective hatred may allow for the restoration of linkages with the sequestered incestuous self. The challenge to the survivor is to locate her hatred before she is known and recognized by the perpetrator. This is the paradox of the perpetrator-survivor relation in which each partner requires the prior recognition of the other in order to restore his or her own memory and authentic subjectivity.

## ADHESIVE VIOLATION OF THE OTHER: CAMUS'S *THE STRANGER*

In order to penetrate the phenomenological state of felt innocence in a condition of actual guilt, it is important to live, temporarily, inside the state of "adhesive" dissociation: in its moment-to-moment autohypnotic shifts; in the riveting and haunting power of sybaritic excess to momentarily annihilate or awaken, but to ultimately leave one empty and without an interior; in the simultaneity of flattening, somnolent deadness and hyperalert acuity to detail; in the elasticity of time; in the isolation and alienation of the soul from the body; in the inexplicable floods of sensation, image, and affect; in the loss of the sense of agency for one's acts. Life is a desperate struggle for equilibrium; the threat of unfelt terror is absolute and surrender impossible. The other does not exist. I agree with Mitrani (1994b) that the fullest phenomenological analysis of such states may be found in literature.[2]

Camus's (1955) novel *The Stranger* allows us to live inside this state in the character of Meursault. Camus's story is simple. In this narrative, we enter and remain in the existential present. Meursault is a man who lives without history and without memory. He lives

---

2. Camus's (1955) own avowed intention is at variance with my interpretation of the novel. But the fit is so remarkable, I can only question whether there is a dissociated quality to Camus's existentialist position as articulated in *The Stranger*.

an ordinary life in Algiers. He receives word that his mother has died. He attends the wake and the funeral for a day; he returns home and begins a liaison with Marie, becomes embroiled in Raymond's affair of passion, and, in the course of a day at the beach, commits a senseless and passionless murder for which he is tried and convicted and sentenced to death.

Meursault is the central character of this novel, set in a landscape suffused with brilliant light shimmering on white sand and blue water. He is an alienated sensualist for whom life has no meaning or significance beyond the immediate hedonic pleasure of sun and sea and a woman's caress. He initiates nothing, he intends nothing; he is without feelings or attachments. He has no interior. Our perspective as reader is a remarkable one: as he is our narrator we are taken inside him, and yet, there is no inside of him to enter. We have been taken inside of nothingness. Meursault lives in continually shifting dissociative states of numbness, unreality, and remoteness; a mere witness to the events of his life. Although he appears to live for the body he is never *embodied*; he never possesses a lived and related self located in his bodily experience. For Meursault, there is no subjective self and there is no human other.

Meursault's autohypnotic and depersonalized states are regulated by the shifting sensations of light and heat, by the play of light on sand and water, by the sounds of water trickling and of insects humming. Insofar as there is an other in his autistic sensory universe, it is the living and capricious African sun that dominates his world. The whiteness of the sand, the yellow haze of the sun, and the blue of the water are the body of Meursault's eternal lover. His life is lived in pursuit of the perfect sensory conditions that will create his "psychic skin" and allow him moments of exhilarating aliveness. But the sun has many moods: at one moment it offers a soft warm caress and a soothing lethargy; at another a menacing, relentless, and disintegrative heat. This is an inescapable sun, which illuminates and blinds, awakens and deadens, nurtures and destroys.

We perceive Meursault much as he perceives the landscape: as a brilliantly illuminated surface, devoid of hidden recess, of subtlety and shadow, of interiority. It is a landscape in which the sun is absolute, without either the comfort or pain of darkness. When black objects occasionally appear on the landscape, shimmering in the sun, mute and impenetrable, they are not-to-be-known. They seem to represent the dissociated black hole against which Meursault anaesthetizes himself; they frequently presage a shift into somnolent withdrawal: "In front, the coachman's glossy black hat looked like a lump of some sticky substance, poised above the hearse. It gave one a queer dreamlike impression, that blue white glare overhead and all this blackness round one: the sleek black of the hearse, the dull black of the men's clothes and the silvery-black gashes in the road . . . what with these . . . I found my eyes and thoughts growing blurred" (p. 20). Only once does he allow himself to recognize the comfort of encountering the darkness, while at his mother's funeral procession: "Evenings in these parts must be a sort of mournful solace. Now, in the full glare of the morning sun, with everything shimmering in the heat haze, there was something inhuman, discouraging, about this landscape" (p. 18).

Meursault will not voluntarily enter the darkness, which would potentiate his own subjectivity; he adheres to the flat surface of heat and light. But the black hole will find him because, for Meursault, there is no authentic containment, no inside or outside, no self and other. Others exist as sources of sensation or a means to pass the time. They are without animation. At his mother's wake, Meursault describes the others present who are able to weep for his mother: "Never in my life had I seen anyone so clearly as I saw these people; not a detail of their clothes or features escaped me. And yet, I couldn't hear them, and it was hard to believe they really existed" (p. 10). Here Camus conveys to us the dissociative hyperacuity for sensory detail, and the simultaneous sense that no one is truly human or really real. Meursault cannot grasp the sense of human connectedness revealed to him through their tears; he can only witness others' grief from a remote and indifferent stance of numbness and oblivion. It is evident to everyone present that he *did not know her*; he neither loved nor hated her; he cannot even say how old she was when she died. He experiences only a remote guilt for missing a day at the office, and a mild preference for a day at the beach. This indifference to others' humanity, as well as his

utter lack of affect and attachment, permeates his relations with
both his friend Raymond and his lover Marie as well.

This dim core of nothingness and the unfelt nameless dread of
not-being moves him, inexorably, toward the annihilation of the
inanimate other: the murder of the Arab. Raymond has beaten his
mistress, the Arab's sister, for infidelity. The Arab is waiting for
Raymond one day at the beach. There is an altercation; Meursault
is an inert, numb witness. Raymond is cut; Raymond and
Meursault retreat to the beach house. While Raymond attends to
his wounds, Meursault embarks for another walk on the beach to
escape the oppressive heat in the house. It is no better on the
beach. He continues to walk, without thought or intention, and
discovers himself at the same spot where the Arab had been. He
has vaguely assumed the Arab would be gone. The heat and light
are relentless, inescapable. He enters a desperate field of sensory
disintegration and overstimulation that hurls him towards psychic
death. His second skin is shattered by the clanging and roaring of
a thousand piercing refractions of light and scalding heat. It is a
moment without memory or intention. Past and future collapse in
a desperate tropic movement to escape sensory annihilation; his
hand moves on the trigger.

The Arab is a dark blur, a lifeless *thing*, no different dead or
alive: an incidental pawn in Meursault's reprieve from the black
hole of nonbeing. He is murdered without hatred and without
desire. The hand that pulls the trigger is not *really real* or really
Meursault's. Even as another self hears the cataclysmic crack of
gunfire, Meursault is absent. He witnesses neither the death nor
the dying, reawakening to consciousness in prison. He is mildly
puzzled at being treated like a criminal. Although technically he
"knows" that he has committed murder, he experiences himself
as an innocuous botanic trope: innocent, ordinary, protoplasmic.
When the judge asks him why he committed the murder, he can
only say, truthfully, *because of the sun*. It is for this response, and for
smoking and drinking coffee at his mother's wake, that he is condemned to death. He is condemned not so much for the murder,
but for his indifferent, dead, and remorseless state; for the utter
bankruptcy of his object relatedness.

Meursault begins to awaken from his dissociative haze when he meets the "objective hatred" of those who condemn him. At one moment during the trial he cries his only tear because, "I felt a sort of wave of indignation spreading through the courtroom, and for the first time, I understood that I was guilty" (p. 112). His act is becoming really *real*, really *his* and really *murder* only as he approaches the scaffold. In his confrontation with the priest he has his first impassioned, object-related encounter. He rages at the priest for his offer of religious illusion to comfort him in his imminent death. In his rage, Meursault has at last entered the painful exaltation of the real; he has found volition. He repudiates the priest's sleep of illusion even as he faces the ultimate and final darkness. Meursault is alive, embodied, and he is at last able to feel loneliness. Because he still cannot feel remorse for the Arab, he must die. All he can do is to make his own death fully alive. "For all to be accomplished, for me to feel less lonely, all that remained to hope was that on the day of my execution there should be a huge crowd of spectators and that they should greet me with howls of execration" (p. 154). It is their continued object-related rage that will render him human and less alone even as he is dying. He will "rage against the dying of the light," meeting passion with passion, allowing the murderer within him to be seen and known even as it has already begun its transformation.

Camus has offered us a brilliant phenomenology of the autistic world of dissociative sensation as he traces Meursault's inexorable path toward murder. He offers us an "adhesive" perpetrator self who commits a solipsistic crime without knowledge or volition, memory or desire. *The Stranger* illustrates the conviction of innocence in a condition of actual guilt. In its final scenes, we see that the perpetrator's dawning emergence from autistic depersonalization into the realm of self and other is realized only in the moment when he finally meets the "objective hatred" of societal condemnation. This emergence holds within it the potential for the development of depressive remorse and mutuality. For Meursault, as for the "adhesive" perpetrator, it is possible to begin his awakening only on the scaffolds of objective hatred.

# CHAPTER 5

# MALIGNANCE AND THE BESTIALITY
# OF SURVIVAL

❦

BARELY 20 YEARS OLD, THEY WERE ORPHANS IN A STRANGE CITY.
They were in love, but their love was a destructive enmeshment.
Sarah had just suggested separation. He was desolate and abandoned; he had no one else. She was guilty and confused. He was
murdered that very night. She too, was meant to be murdered. She
survived, but she was debased by her own courage.

That evening, they drank wine in a city park. A stranger took
them to his apartment. There was beer, and then a request for
pornographic photos of her. They said no. Now everything hap-
pens in an eternal present. The stranger takes out a gun. As the gun
moves towards her lover's head, Sarah sees a look of resigned desolation in his eyes. In this resignation she reads his response to her
imminent abandonment. He does not move, does not fight or
struggle. Quietly he says, "I guess this is the end of my life." There
is a blast, the room is awash with blood, his corpse lies on the
floor. There is another blast and a bullet grazes her head. She is
bleeding.

Unlike her lover, she is neither immobile nor resigned. She
finds herself alive, and she wants to stay alive. And so, she enters the
murderer's interior and offers herself as his accomplice, a murderer
like himself. She pretends to have felt nothing for her lover, to
have barely known him, not to care that he has been murdered.
She has no intention of going to the police. She complies with sex

in full view of her lover's corpse, and pretends to like it. Sex over, she discusses plans for the disposal of the body, for the murderer's concealment. She plans "their" escape. She washes the blood from the murderer's clothes. She bandages and conceals her own wound. They dispose of the corpse, dragging its bulk down an abandoned stairwell, as if it were so much illicit refuse. The murderer is cold, flat, monosyllabic. Together they get on a bus, with the intent to get away. She gets off at the next stop, and miraculously, he does not detain her. She has induced him to trust her. She goes to the police, leads them to the body, then to the bus depot. The murderer is caught, and prosecuted. She testifies and he is condemned. He is never prosecuted for rape because, in her compliance, she can show no bruises, no evidence of struggle. In the eyes of "justice," the threat of murder does not constitute a sufficient display of force.

It would take 10 years of treatment before she could know herself as a rape victim. It would take 15 years of treatment before she could know herself as loving, courageous. What she knew, what she lived, was the sheer brutality of her own survival: her culpability, her guilt, her incapacity for love. She did not throw herself across the body of her beloved. She did not die in protest. She had sex with the man who murdered her lover; she dragged her beloved's body to the bottom of an abandoned stairwell. She had precipitated her lover's suicidal immobility. Perhaps she had even wanted him dead. She was complicit in murder and felt that she had forfeited all innocence.

For many years, she pursued the death which she should have died. She pursued it in infinite permutations of self-abuse and endangerment. And in an endless recapitulation of the murder, the moment of her death always eluded her, averted by the tenacity of her capacity for survival.

Psychotherapy articulated her wordless enactments, and ameliorated her sense of badness. She lived a good life. But ultimately, it was only in supreme existential penance that she could approach innocence and separation. It was 30 years later. She had tenderly nursed her current lover through cancer and comforted him in his death. She had nursed her sister through cancer, and mourned her death. Even as her sister lay dying, Sarah almost died of cancer her-self. She endured the scourge of chemotherapy. Her job was "downsized" and she was unemployed. She was suddenly destitute, while attempting to manage enormous medical expenses. She sought work while depleted by illness and by grief. In her own life, she met each crisis with dignity, never failing herself or others in any human gesture.

In its perversity, life had provided her with an opportunity that psychotherapy could only approximate. Her capacity for survival was now suffused with an experience of her own goodness. At last, she had her first dream of innocence. She dreamed of saying a benign goodbye to her young lover. In this goodbye, his solitude and his despair had dissipated; he was drunk, but he knew a desire to live. It was a youthful breakup, repossessed of youth's simplicity and resilience. They would both go on living. In the wake of this dream, there is a new calm and a new beginning. Her memories of the murder now carry an awakened knowledge of her own lov-ing courage and pursuit of justice. Nonetheless, the knowledge of her own strength will always be attended by an awareness of her own dark possibilities.

## TERROR, BESTIALITY, AND THE ETHICS OF SURVIVAL

In conditions of terror and oppression, the fullness of the victim's ethical integrity is rarely sustained unless she quickly succumbs to death. When death is not swift, the victim must live in negotiation with the imminence of annihilation. To live in anticipation of extinction is to experience moments of extraordinary humanity; but it is also to succumb to primitive imperatives. In the urgency of survival, courage and ruthlessness become inseparable. For, as Amery (1995) suggests, one is "Frail in the face of violence, yelling out in pain, awaiting no help, capable of no resistance, the tortured person is only a body" (p. 131). In this state, survival is an act of courage; but it is also a reduction to flesh. As Langer (1991) would suggest, survival invariably entails a moment of ethical collapse in which the self or the other (or both) is morally betrayed. In survival's last extremity, the mind repudiates such betrayal, and the body compels that which the mind refuses. The mind becomes the antagonist of the body, and the body's desire for life is confounded with an experienced moral transgression. When the survivor is forced to violate her own ethical code, when she acts in base opposition to her honor, she has engaged in the *bestial gesture of survival.*

In this chapter, I suggest that the victim's bestial gesture fulfills the soul murderer's intentions: it reduces the victim to nothing but a body-it, devoid of freedom (Sartre, 1956); it extinguishes the victim's essential goodness, which the sadist envies and must destroy (McGinn,1997), and it allows the perpetrator to elude accountability. As a body-it, the victim is broken. And as a body-it, she can neither accuse nor remember. One must be human to accuse and to remember. In survival, it is the guilty self that remains human, and it is the guilty self that survives to accuse and remember. But accusation is largely turned against the self in atonement for the bestial gesture. Here, the "masochist feels like a criminal, and the psychopathic sadist feels like a victim" (Howell, 1996, p. 427). This transaction is an essential aspect of the perpetrator's "brutality of spirit and . . . exaltation of power" (Waite, 1952, p. 281). In its wake, the perpetrator has succeeded in forcing the victim to *want* death (McGinn, 1997) for having wanted life.

To refuse the victimizer's intentions, psychoanalysis must evolve an intrapsychic and intersubjective analysis of the survivor's felt experience of ethical transgression. This chapter is therefore devoted to an analysis of bestial guilt and bestial memory. In particular, I investigate the survivor's experience of *wanting death for having wanted life.* Often, the survivor seeks death and self-immolation, unconsciously pursuing an idealized heroic death. What is the meaning and significance of this suicidal desire? How does it simultaneously construct and deconstruct evil's relational matrix? I will propose that the desire for death derives from a nascent depressive subjectivity. Upon analysis, we find that the death that is desired is a transcendent death, in which an intact depressive subject refuses to surrender her ethical integrity.

In honoring the nobility and refusal inherent in the survivor's suicidal desire, the analyst acknowledges that the survivor possesses "an inner split which is both guilty and deadly" (Lifton, 1996, p. 131). Such an analyst does not simply seek to ameliorate the survivor's excessive sense of badness. Rather, the analyst respects the narrative of the patient's guilty memory, recognizing that it is "fruitless . . . to contradict a patient who brings these accusations against his ego. He must surely be right in some way. . . . He has lost his self respect and he must have good reason for this." (Freud, 1925, pp. 146–147). The analyst comprehends guilt and despair as an *insatiable reparative hunger that seeks love's reparative effectance*. She seeks to empower guilt rather than to simply eradicate it, knowing that, as A. Williams (1998) suggests, recovery from persecutory anxiety may require a real reparative act. Indeed, as Mitchell (1993a) notes, "Only by embracing one's destructiveness can one transcend it through forgiveness and reparation towards real others, internal objects, and ultimately, the self" (p. 381).

Thus, I contextualize my analysis of the survivor's bestial gesture in the language of the depressive modality: in terms of guilt, in terms of reparative versus manic defense; and in terms of object-related hatred and concern. I suggest that the victim's ethical transgression organizes and *dis*organizes reparative and manic defenses. Here, either good *or* evil can be potentiated. Insofar as the survivor wants death for having wanted life, goodness is potentiated; insofar as the survivor has foreclosed all reparative longing, evil is potentiated.

## THE PHENOMENOLOGY OF THE BESTIAL EXCHANGE

The bestial gesture is a marriage of toxicity and desire. Through it, the victim's life force is confounded with the destructive force "that continues after . . . it destroys existence, time and space" (Bion, 1965, p. 101). The life force has forever lost the purity of innocence, the joy that should reside in bodily desire:

Blackness filled me, spread from the back of my head into my eyes as if my brain had been punctured. Spread from stomach to legs, I gulped and gulped, swallowing it whole. The wall filled with smoke. I struggled out and stared while the air caught fire.

I wanted to go to my parents, to touch them. But I couldn't, unless I stepped on their blood.

The soul leaves the body instantly, as if it can hardly wait to be free: my mother's face was not her own. My father was twisted with falling. Two shapes in the flesh-heap, his hands . . .

I ran . . .

Then I felt the worst shame of my life: I was pierced with hunger [Michaels, 1997, pp. 7–9].

Here, the command of hunger severs this fictional boy from the loyalty of his sorrow. How can he desire bread? The desire for bread is a soulless desire; it severs his life from familial love and from the memory of familial murder. He feels that his hunger renders him as cold as their murderer. He should be paralyzed with grief. And still, it is bread that compels him. In his pursuit of life, he imagines himself justly orphaned from humanity: "So hungry. I screamed into the silence the only phrase I knew in more than one language, I screamed it in Polish and German and Yiddish, thumping my fists on my own chest: dirty Jew, dirty Jew, dirty Jew" (Michaels, 1997, pp. 12–13).

The survivor's sense of being justly orphaned from humanity is often derived from such poignant verbal or bodily gestures. It occurs wherever the oppressed are forced to collude in their own oppression. Even the survivor who has demonstrated great moral fortitude is haunted by some experienced ethical violation. For Winston in *1984* (Orwell, 1949), it is his cry, "Do it to Julia." In incest, it may be located in the contradiction between the mind's disgust and the body's arousal (Ehrenberg, 1987; Lionells, 1992). During African-American slavery, it may have been the slave's coerced, mendacious defense of his master's "kindness," even as the slave bore the scar of the master's whippings upon his back

(Douglass, 1845). For gays and lesbians, it may have been the public pretense of heterosexuality, and the tolerance of homophobic comments. For Sarah, it was the "victimless crime" of concealing her lover's corpse. At other times, the transgression is truly a transgression. In Pol Pot's regime a torture device was constructed to decapitate children attempting to escape from prison camps, and *other children, themselves threatened with this torture and death, were forced to operate this device* (*Time*, August 18, 1997).

Thus, the bestial gesture may entail a real act of betrayal, exploitation, violence, in which victims are forced to commit heinous acts to survive. It may entail a relatively benign feeling, thought, or bodily function that the victim *experiences* as a moral transgression against the self or others. It may occur in adulthood or childhood. In some instances, the experienced transgression is largely a matter of fantasy. Insofar as the transgression is a reality, these realities are characterized by varying degrees of coercion and moral agency; they are differentially responsive to healing and to self-forgiveness, and they dictate different therapeutic strategies. Nonetheless, these moments share a certain resonance: they signify the marriage between ethical collapse and primitive desire; they precipitate guilt and reparative hunger. And they compel the survivor to want death for wanting life.

If survival is inevitably marked by moral violation and a quest for atonement, so it is inevitably imbued with a dissociative inability to establish the *historical locus of horror*. Here the perpetrator locates his greatest triumph and concealment: the true history of the perpetrator's culpability is occluded in the survivor's shared monstrosity. Indeed, it is through the bestial gesture that the "shadow of the object falls upon the ego" (Freud, 1925), and the perpetrator's guilt inhabits the survivor's soul. Who is culpable? Who must be penitent? It is a tribute to the perpetrator's brilliance that the survivor's coerced transgression obscures questions of agency and responsibility, guilt and innocence. In the survivor's breach of his own moral integrity, the perpetrator locates a mirror for his own disavowed culpability. In Auschwitz, for example, the commandant Hoss (1946) watched prisoners feeding off other prisoners, forcing each other into gas chambers, searching the dead for food, dragging the bodies of friends and relatives to the crematoriums. He considered such activities in the vacuum of his own agency, remarking on the prisoners' inhumanity as if they were free to refuse. These observations supported his contention that Jews were subhuman and thus required extermination. His achievement of forcing prisoners to collude in their own physical and moral extinction remains invisible in his autobiography. He observes the female capos' sadism:

> They far surpassed their male equivalents in toughness, squalor, vindictiveness and depravity. Most were prostitutes with many convictions, and some were truly repulsive creatures. Needless to say, these dreadful women gave full vent to their evil desires on the prisoners under them. . . . They were soulless and had no feelings whatsoever. . . . I find it incredible that human beings could ever turn into such beasts. The way the "greens" knocked the French Jewesses about, tearing them to pieces, killing them with axes, and throttling them—it was simply gruesome [Hoss, 1946, pp. 76–77].

For Hoss, the depraved actions of the prisoners were not precipitated by his own cruelty. Rather, such actions demonstrated that it was the Jews, not the Nazis, who were responsible for the real acts of sadism in Auschwitz: "They were mainly persecuted by members of their own race, their foremen or room seniors" (Hoss, 1946, p. 70). By contrast, Hoss considered himself responsible for the regrettable but necessary extinction of unwanted segments of humanity. His own efforts at *humane* extinction were frustrated in the unfortunate chaos of the war years. He perceived himself as a troubled but hardened victim of civic duty, a man who never hated Jews, a thoughtful aesthete who appreciated his Auschwitz home as a "paradise of flowers" (Hoss, 1946, p. 107).

This, then, is the perversity of survival: that victim and perpetrator are inextricably linked through the survivor's bestial gesture. The victim is haunted by her own moral failure, and the perpetrator is cleansed and obscured in the survivor's guilt. For Sarah, this metaphor is concretized in the washing of the perpetrator's blood from his clothes: the evidence of his culpability dissolves in the inhuman acts of her survival. To Sarah, the worst betrayal and violation was her own: *he* merely murdered a stranger; *she* violated and betrayed a loved one. She does more "time" than the murderer in his cell. And what of him, in his cell? One can imagine him as one imagines Hoss: caged and remorseless, endlessly cataloguing his own victimization.

## TERROR, BESTIALITY, AND THE COLLAPSE OF THE DEPRESSIVE SUBJECT

### The Depressive Modality

How can psychoanalysts restructure this inversion of accusation and accountability? To interrupt the perpetrator's concealment, we must penetrate the unconscious meaning of bestial mutual influence. To do so, we must turn to an understanding of the depressive collapse that occurs in trauma. We must first comprehend the "normal" depressive struggle: the surrender of narcissistic omnipotence, the birth of empathy and responsibility, the evolution of "creative" (Winnicott, 1954, 1958, 1963) guilt and concern, the awareness of loss, and the awakening of grief. We then become able to examine the ways in which annihilation and bestial transformation disorganize that depressive struggle, thereby potentiating *and refusing* malignant dissociative contagion.

Beginning with Freud's (1925) description of object loss, mourning and melancholia, Klein (1946), Winnicott (1954, 1963), Riviere, (1964), Segal (1964), and Ogden (1989), have articulated a "depressive" mode of being. This mode is critical to the evolution of a truly "moral" character. It is characterized by a genuine, empathic sensitivity to the other, and by the birth of interpersonal moral responsibility: there is a new capacity to comprehend one's own hurtful potential, to experience authentic remorse, and to

seek opportunities to make amends to the object of the transgression. At the same time, a new kind of hate evolves: an ability
to hate the other's destructiveness, and to nonetheless view this
destructive other as *human*. This depressive hate impels a pursuit
of justice and containment, rather than vengeance. As will become
evident below, all of these capacities follow upon a singular developmental achievement: the recognition of self and other as separate centers of experience (see Benjamin, 1999), linked in a
relation of potential intimacy and potential loss.

Like Freud, Klein and the neo-Kleinians emphasize the role of
object loss in the development of the depressive position or modality. Unlike Freud, they do not focus on the narcissistic fusion with
the lost object; rather, they study the interaction of destruction,
object loss, and self–other differentiation. For Ogden, Klein, Riviere,
Segal, and Winnicott, the very hallmark of the depressive modality
is self–other differentiation. Where infancy was characterized by an
imaginary merger with the other, a grandiose omnipotence, and by
the wanton use of the other, there is now an ambivalent understanding that the other exists outside of the self. That other is gradually recognized as a separate human *subject*, possessed of her own
vulnerable interior, a figure who can be injured, lost, perhaps never
to be regained. There is a new recognition that the self is not
omnipotent, but rather, is dependant upon another *who may or may
not be there*. The anticipation of loss is not a passively held position;
rather it is agentic. In the depressive mode, loss is understood as precipitated by one's own destructive capacity. There is a sudden awareness that the wanton use of the other may have created an
irreparable "hole" in the other's psyche/soma (Winnicott, 1954).
Grief, despair, and guilt awaken, engendering an urgent need to
reconstitute a loving relation through the repair of the other. This
need is what Klein, Segal, and Winnicott call the *desire to make reparation*. It is through true guilt (Winnicott, 1958, 1963) and reparative
effectance that the other is restored and one's own mourning and
despair are ameliorated. And, as Odgen (1989) suggests, it is through
the establishment of this depressive subjectivity that one evolves a
capacity to know one's own history: to know the past as continu-

ous, interpretable, and nonetheless immutable. Thus, the empathic I–Thou relation of reparative effectance is coextensive with the maintenance of the historical, symbolic self.

Insofar as one's interpersonal field offers opportunities for reparation, one is possessed of reparative effectance. Guilt is not transformed into pathological masochism and depression. Instead, guilt is an affirmative, generative experience. It has a creative (Winnicott, 1954) or animating (Lifton, 1996) function that contributes to a sense of social responsibility (Lifton, 1996), goodness, and creativity (Klein, 1948; Klein and Riviere, 1964; Segal, 1964). Even as individuation and agentic guilt give birth to the intersubjective intimacy of mutual recognition (Benjamin, 1988), so they give birth to the capacity for "object-related hatred" (Winnicott, 1947). Even as the beloved, damaged other can be seen and restored, so the destructive subjective other can now be known and recognized through containing hatred. This hate is not the fractured, dehumanizing hate of the paranoid–schizoid modality, in which one's vision of the real other is occluded by the mechanisms of splitting and projection. Depressive hate entails a real meeting with and perception of the other; it involves a restraint of the other's destructiveness. Thus, in the successful depressive struggle, the person evolves twin capacities. She evolves a sense of goodness and reparative effectance in relation to those against whom she has transgressed. And, her historical self becomes able to see, know, and contain the other's destructiveness.

Where the intersubjective context fails to provide opportunities for reparative effectance, the twin capacities for object-related concern and hatred are attenuated. "Animated" guilt collapses into an abyss of mourning and self-blame; the symbolic, agentic, historical self is unborn. For some, depressive subjectivity is in a state of becoming: it makes its evolving presence known through an excess of guilt and depression. For others, empathic depressive subjectivity is foreclosed through the manic defense. In the "manic" defense, the individual takes flight from experiencing the dependency needs that are felt to precipitate loss, guilt, mourning, and despair. Rather than experiencing dependency needs and their attendant depressive conflicts, this person denies her own guilt and despair. She utilizes splitting and projective identification to locate affective need and vulnerability outside of the self, then disdaining and annihilating others. This defensive structure becomes characterological cruelty and contempt (Klein and Riviere, 1964; Segal, 1964).

From this perspective, we begin to comprehend the pivotal role that reparation holds in ordinary moral and intersubjective development. We also begin to comprehend the role that reparation plays in the attainment of *historical subjectivity: that capacity to know history as simultaneously interpretable and nonetheless immutable.* And we can understand how life's pedestrian depressive struggle is eclipsed by *real* annihilation and by the survivor's sense of moral transgression. In the wake of the bestial gesture, the need to repair the other is exponentially increased, even as the reparative capacity has received a cataclysmic blow. In the bestial moment, the victim's desire for life has caused an irreparable wound in the psyche/soma of the self, the other, or both. It is a hole so deep, a silence so absolute, that it cannot be fully healed even by the most robust reparative capacity. Thus the moral transgression of survival articulates an outer limit of reparative possibility. The impossibility of reparative restoration is often concretized in the real death or disappearance of those against whom one has transgressed (Sarah's lover). And the self who would make reparation has been vanquished: at the very moment when the reparative capacity must demonstrate superhuman effectance, it has been intentionally eviscerated by the perpetrator. The ethical transgression of survival therefore precipitates depressive collapse. There is a regression from the depressive position that "manifests itself in survivor guilt, which represents internalization of the original Nazi aggressor. The superego now threatens the survivor with the same extermination that threatened him in the concentration camps. Survivor guilt also represents a link to the dead" (Bergmann, 1985, p. 18).

The fragmentary remains of the depressive self are left with a sense of reparative impotence and reparative longing. This constitutes an insatiable hunger: it causes the survivor to *want death for having wanted life.*

## *Reparative Hunger and the Death of the Depressive Self*

In the theater of survivors' lives, in the interior of their fantasies and dreams, we witness this masochistic pull toward self-destruction (Bergmann, 1985; Courtois, 1988; Herman 1992; Waites, 1993; Alpert, 1994; Davies and Frawley, 1994). For years after the murder, Sarah drunkenly surrenders her body to strange men. They beat her. She awakens to the imprint of their sex upon her body. And still, she is not dead. She gets drunk again, seeking situations of increasing danger. Later, we understand these enactments as a pursuit of the death that she should have died. She seeks a death of ethical integrity, in which she no longer survives through the betrayal of her beloved.

Like many survivors, Sarah feels that, in survival, " 'We must carry each other. If we don't have this, what are we'" (Michaels, 1997, p. 14). We must carry others and ourselves in dignity, in humanity, in ethical integrity. Like every survivor, she holds a vision of a victim who carries herself forward into death in an act of grace. We get a sense of such imagery as we listen to Nazi commandant Hoss as he supervises the gassing of Jews in Auschwitz:

> One young woman caught my attention particularly as she ran busily hither and thither, helping the smallest children and the old women to undress. During the selection she had had two small children with her, and her agitated behavior and appearance had brought her to my notice at once. She did not look the least like a Jewess. Now her children were no longer with her. She waited until the end, helping the women who were not undressed and who had several children with them, encouraging them and calming the children. She went with the very last ones into the gas-chamber. Standing in the doorway, she said: "I knew all the time that we were being brought to Auschwitz to be gassed. When the selection took place I avoided being put with the able-bodied ones, as I wished to look after the children. Goodbye" [Hoss, 1946, pp. 99–100].

The sight of terrorized innocents and the dignified courage of this woman failed to move Hoss from his "necessary, but regrettable task" of mass annihilation (Hoss, 1946). And yet, an ordinary woman meets her extinction in full possession of her own humanity, inscribing her courage even on those Nazis who witness it. It is a death that survivors have escaped, but it is a death of which they may well be covetous. For it appears to be a death of untrammeled integrity, in which the body is extinguished but the soul survives. Paradoxically, this self is imagined to transcend death even as it surrenders.

In this idealized refusal to relinquish her own ethical subjectivity, the impossible appears to become possible. It is almost as if the original moment of annihilation can become populated by "like subjects" (Benjamin, 1995); the perpetrator must surely awaken to his shame and to his defeat. The perpetrator's depressive awakening can appear imminent; perhaps evil will reach its terminus. The woman in Auschwitz does appear humanized in Hoss's memory, her history lives, we can still hear her voice. And yet, of course, intersubjective recognition has never transpired: she has never been known; his acts are never arrested by guilt and concern. Ultimately, the significance of her death is eradicated: because she possesses honor, "She did not look the least like a Jewess" (Hoss, 1946, p. 99). And although she is both honorable and not *really* Jewish, she is still not a "like subject" (Benjamin, 1995). The gas chamber doors can still be sealed behind her. Nonetheless, in the survivor's fantasy, the reparative death promises to command recognition in the executioner. Indeed, although it does not arrest the execution, it nevertheless defeats the perpetrator's pleasure in the breaking of one's soul.

As psychoanalysts, we can understand this dignified death as a death *lived* by the historical depressive subject. It appears to be soulful, empathic, fully possessed of memory and of history, ontologically secure even in extinction. It is *object-related*, aroused in protest, yet fully empowered to make human reparation in the face of the greatest evil. The victim is no longer subjugated in bestiality. Instead, the reparative death reverses the abysmal core of the bestial gesture: the moment when the soul is extinguished, and the body lives on in what Langer (1991) calls "humiliated memory." The attainment of such a death is imagined to subvert evil's ultimate intentions: that is, the moral debasement of the survivor's own interior, and the severing of the survivor's human link. In the shelter of such a death, one never becomes an "it" in the perpetrator's universe. Freedom is never extinguished and the survivor is never reduced to flesh (Sartre, 1956). One never becomes the body-it, who can neither accuse nor remember. In "choosing death before dishonor," the victim remains the subject of her own desire (Benjamin, 1988). She knows her cohorts in empathic concern even as she knows her perpetrator in objective hatred. She dies in a state of integrated surrender, averting her own annihilation by *choosing* her own death. She is now free: she is no longer forced to want death for having wanted life; she seeks death because it *restores* life.

## ANALYSIS AS A THEATER OF CRUELTY AND SURVIVAL

As an analyst, I have found myself wanting death for having wanted life. At the time I treated Donna, I was ill, and I wanted to stay alive. She met my illness with an unmitigated cruelty. Gradually, I came to know her as the agent of my bodily destruction. I sensed that only my death could infuse her with life. And so, my illness became the real life precipitant of a countertransference enactment from which I have never entirely recovered (see Hirsch, 1993). For I discovered this: that during a serious illness, the analyst can become prey to both a "maximum attack on her subjectivity" (Benjamin, 1999), and to a maximum attack on her bodily integrity (see also Schlesinger-Silver, 1990; Schwartz, 1990). At such times, the metaphoric field of analysis (Schwartz, 1990) collapses, and the threat of *real* annihilation must be negotiated. For me, this involved a "collapse of the space in which it is possible to think" (Benjamin, 1999, p. 203). There was no thought, there was no reflection, no "recognizing third" position (Ogden, 1994) between us. It was a simple field without the intervening space of metaphor: her life and my death *or* her death and my life. Here was my bestial gesture of survival: I was enclosed in my own dread and could offer no mutual escape from our affliction. I secured my own life and compromised her infant self. Sometimes, I think that she would have located any analyst's dread. Perhaps induced dread was the only arena in which her infant self could speak. I am almost innocent. It is a brief reprieve. In truth, it was impossible for me to bear her vindictiveness (see Feiner, 1995) and locate her murdered infant self while I was in a state of psychic dissolution. But she herself was an agent of that dissolution.

In psychoanalysis, we neither speak nor write of our own transgressions. Only our patients know of them, and often they dare not, cannot, speak. In our silence, we pose as a discipline without failures, a human discourse without terror, a collective mind that is not subject to the parameters of death. We foreclose our guilt, as well as all access to reparation and redemption. And we exempt ourselves from the human condition. And so, in the presentation of this case, I invite analysts to admit that we are not exempt.

## THE CASE OF DONNA

I think of her often. I find myself culpable. I find myself innocent. I need some form of address, some answering resonance. Writing it is a confessional, a search for absolution, but it is a stone cast into stagnant water. Rather than surrender to solitude, I would submit to judgment. But even in the possibility of judgment, solitude is not ameliorated. Perhaps the truth of this story is that it is a story bereft of answering resonance. It is always changing, always possessed of another meaning, never finite, never still, never fully lived in relation to another. I can never reach her, and she is never known.

It was 10 years ago, perhaps more. For two years prior to meeting Donna, I had suffered severe and recurrent infections, becoming increasingly unresponsive to antibiotic treatment. Previously I had been robust. I was young. I had not really thought of dying. Now, my immune system was mysteriously suppressed. Doctors treated each infection, but promised nothing. It was inexplicable.

I had not had either AIDS or cancer. I had been well, and now I was ill. At times, my patients arrived for their sessions coughing, sneezing, complaining of fever. In the ordinariness of their colds I found a grimmer threat. I thought: next time, I'll die of it, and they'll survive.

I survived these times, offering my patients my "intact" therapeutic self, unapproachable in the area of my illness. I felt that to be seen by my patients as a sick person would have been an invasion of the privacy of my dread. Their knowledge would implode (Laing, 1960) the delicate restitution of my interior, an interior lost in the failed bodily boundary of immunity. For in the failure of my immunity, insides had flooded into outsides, and outsides into insides. I longed for an impermeable border between inside and outside, between contagion and resistance. I needed to locate an inviolable perimeter for death.

And so, my patients loved me by articulating my insides and outsides, by cocreating an impermeable border, a metaphorical barrier of immunity. Together we defined my outsides and they remained "outside" of me. They loved me by using me as an intact analyst; by failing to notice my ashen skin, my weight loss, the pattern of my absences. They knew me by allowing me to hold my illness and my own madness in privacy and seclusion. Instead, they located, used, and reawakened my remaining empathic strength, covertly recognizing me as a subject-in-dread by overtly using me as an illusory intact *object*. In their eyes, I was sane and I was well. They held the states of my fragility and terror in what Ghent (1992) calls, "benign illusion." It was an act of great tenderness and mercy. And they healed as they used me, and as they used me, I healed. Those patients who required holding (see Slochower, 1996) were held in the illusion of their analyst's intact interior, even as I was held in the boundary of their illusion. Paradoxically, our depressive selves were mutually emergent in this manifest collapse of intersubjectivity. The history of our healing was repressed rather than dissociated, available for subsequent analysis.

Gradually I began to convalesce, in part due to their loving provision of a metaphorical immunity. It was at this stage that I began working with Donna. She possessed that schizoid aggression which is insidious, cold, paranoid, and inhuman (Guntrip, 1971). Intelligent, middle-aged, and professional, she volunteered in a hospice with terminal AIDS and cancer patients. Manifestly kind to the point of self abnegation, she sought treatment for sexual difficulties, claiming that her female lover repudiated Donna's advances. Her lover suggested that Donna had sexual and self-esteem "issues" to explore. Donna was a good girl, and she came in compliance. I accepted her into treatment. We worked hard, we had insights, she felt nothing. She always did the "right" thing, but was devoid of any emotive core.

After six months, she developed a cough. After two weeks of this cough, she made the rather bland announcement that she had viral "walking" pneumonia, although she barely felt ill. Manifestly unconcerned about her own health, she induced in me the terror that I had been infected with a potentially lethal infection. I no longer saw her, but rather, my own death. Suddenly I wondered, *How could I have failed to visualize the hospice where she worked: the influx of infection, the slow, steady arrival of death, the failed supplication of immunity*. I had felt the terrors of my own immune collapse, and yet disavowed it. There was no death and disease. I had accepted her into treatment as a denial of my own mortality; the Donna I took into treatment was, like myself, a healer. We were grandiose, she and I. If I had disavowed the prospect of infection, *so she had disavowed her vulnerable self: she had no aperture for infection, no infant self continuously in the process of dying*.

I determined that I would have to telephone her to explain that I was immune-suppressed and that I could not work with her in person until her illness was resolved. This revelation felt like forfeiting my psychic barrier to invasion, at the very moment when infection may have begun its incubation. After this loss of my boundaries, I must lock the door against her toxicity. And so I met with the dark ethics of survival: self-preservation seemed at odds with professional ethics and commitments. Must I displace her needs with my own? I had had two similar dilemmas with other patients regarding my immune vulnerability and each had been managed both therapeutically and compassionately. Surely it was possible to do so with Donna.

I would offer a referral, and if she refused, I would offer her telephone sessions until our predicament was resolved. Perhaps we might remain together, reaching past her numbness to rage and longing. I anticipated her anger, and I desired it. But I expected it to conform to time's continuum, to be present, and then, to be past. And, in parallel time, my exposure to infection would be present, then becoming past. Her body would cease to be infected, and my body would once again find its own convalescent reprieve. She would find an intact analytic object with whom to experience her own authentic affective response.

When I told her, I assured her that I did not have AIDS or cancer, that I was not dying. She began to get angry about my impingement on her. She pursued a course of treatment for her pneumonia and refused a referral. In the interim, she utilized phone sessions. Although conflicted, she returned to my office about three weeks later, having ascertained that she was not ill. She reported a sense of empowerment: she had experienced feeling and sensation as she released her anger. It seemed that we were functioning as analyst and patient. *But I refused to know that nothing was neat and that nothing was held in the containing parameters of our goodness.*

From time to time, she continued to articulate anger at my disruption of her treatment. This intermittent anger was contextualized in an exaggerated concern for, and interest in, my immune suppression. I did not experience myself as met by concern. Rather, I began to realize that I had to rely on her accuracy when she stated that she was not contagious. Here was my first encounter with *real* annihilation: I did not feel *as if* I was relying on a patient for my life; I *was* relying on a patient for my life. If she was wrong, it could kill me. I began to experience her as the wanton carrier of infection. I did not as yet experience her as wanting to kill me, but rather as capable of casually killing through ignorance and self-neglect. Later, I would recall her speaking, with pseudo-concern, of all the deadly infectious diseases she could contract in the hospice. She had insinuated that this incident would not be the last. I refused to hear something she was struggling to tell me: that our danger was present and irremediable; that her hate was murderous, and without cease; and that my abandonment of her was infinite, and had no conclusion. I could not hear her metaphor of an infant dying.

I could not hear her metaphor because I was in search of my own antithesis: I required a wall, solid, immune, unbreachable. She required access, symbiosis, toxic permeability. I was in search of endings and borders and containers. The immutable passage of time lured me with its lengthening distance from infection, incubation, disease. She seemed to know nothing of present, past, future: for her, time was a lethal expanse of abandonment. I would not remain with her in the timelessness of what Laub and Podell (1995) call, trauma's "empty circle," for timelessness and formlessness implied my own extinction. We were lost in our foreclosure of the symbolic, we had no words, only bodies. And our bodies were in combat: she must transmit her toxic substance, and I must refuse it. I received her split-off communication like a fist in my chest: I could be working with her during another incubation period and *never know it until too late. I could always be in the process of being murdered.* I withdrew into the edifice of my own survival and tried to leave my child, voiceless, beyond the wall.

She would not remain beyond the wall. She began to excoriate my claim of immune vulnerability, to insinuate that I was delusional, malingering. I was weak, she was strong. When I spoke to her of her hatred, she attributed it to my madness. When I spoke to her of my abandonment and of the pain of dependency, she attributed it to my madness. Just as I began to feel worn away, she would retreat into quiet periods during which we seemed to have words and analytic possibility. I discovered that Donna's single mother spent long days locked in her own room. As an infant and as a toddler, Donna was left in pools of urine, in foul diapers; with scraps of food and no water. Each night, Donna's affectionate uncle would stop by. She would be briefly awakened to moments of human contact, and then, he would depart for long hours of silence. Disturbed by the neglect of this child, he entreated various relatives to care for Donna during the daytime. They did so inconsistently, impersonally. When Donna was just past three years old, the uncle moved in and mother disappeared altogether for long periods of "treatment." In subsequent years, Donna's mother lived with them. She was withdrawn and socially humiliating, although never overtly abusive. As a teenager, Donna completely repudiated her mother as a psychotic embarassment, identifying exclusively with this kind and self-sacrificing uncle. Donna and I now understood that Donna had a raging and abandoned infant self beneath her numb exterior. And then, the excoriation of my "delusion of immune suppression" would continue, and I knew that I was the mad and abandoning mother.

In another quiet period, we had reframed her lover's sexual rejection and her unwillingness to be seen nude as indicative of the lover's shame and anxiety. Donna gave the appearance of a deepened understanding of her beloved. But in the next session, Donna announced that she had gone home from the last session and yanked open the shower door to expose her lover, nude, helpless, terrorized, and ashamed. Donna had stood and watched as the lover struggled to cover herself, aware that her lover was humiliated, but utterly unmoved. I asked what made her do this when she now knew that her beloved was in a state of fear and shame. Donna shrugged and stated that she had a right to see her lover nude. Indeed, Donna viewed this violation as a legitimate sexual overture; she viewed her lover's retreat as a typical "erotic rejection." In subsequent sessions, inquiry revealed that she was taunting her lover with insinuations of past and prospective infidelities. Donna was indeed faithful, and knew her lover's long-standing humiliation about potential sexual betrayal. I also discovered two memories that Donna held with amusement. At the age of 10, she had urinated in her mother's tea, and had watched as her mother gagged while drinking it. Donna's mother looked confused; Donna felt triumphant. At the age of 12, Donna left fresh excrement in a pile of her mother's clean laundry, with similar sentiments. When her uncle discovered these episodes, he laughed, and did nothing to stop her. In his laughter, this self-sacrificing uncle was transformed, momentarily, into a lively being. Donna could not turn to her mother with her own dependent longings, nor could she reparatively "heal" her mother's emotional illness. But she could create a bond with her uncle *and* restore him to affective life through their mutual torment of the depressed mother.

And so, her warm human rage at her mother's abandonment became consolidated into a cold and remorseless cruelty.

I commented that for Donna, need and abandonment caused terrible pain and gave rise to a rage which then became cruelty. If Donna was unyielding in her coldness toward her lover, she was gravely insulted in relation to me. She attributed my perceptions to my own incompetence. I suggested that her infantile self was likewise met with internal contempt and cruelty. She would not dignify my statement with a response. And, then, in my body, there was another fist in my chest: now I knew I would not be infected through casual neglect, but rather, with sadistic intent. I gently but firmly asked her not to come to session if she had a fever or a congested cough that might be indicative of pneumonia or TB. She responded with little feeling and with manifest compliance. Here was my second experience of ethical transgression: what kind of analyst requires a patient to monitor her own bodily and affective states and to remove herself from the analysis so as not to destroy the analyst? But then, what type of analyst allows a patient to arrive with a loaded gun? My guilt was equaled by my desire to survive. I knew that I must meet and contain her sadism so that she might reach the desolation and desire hidden in her infant self. I knew that I must contain her sadism if I were to function as her analyst. Still, I wondered, am I containing or exploiting her by telling her not to come with a cough? I think it is both, and I tell no one.

A week later, Donna arrived at a session with a serious congested cough and a 102 degree fever. On entering the session she insinuated that she might have pneumonia, and commented that she knew she wasn't supposed to come in but she didn't care. She indicated considerable pride in her own stoicism as contrasted with my self-indulgent malingering. I drew her attention to her contempt. She stated that she wanted to expose me to getting sick; she wanted to prove to me that my claims of immune suppression were no more than a hypochondriacal delusion. Now I knew the hate that endures in annihilation's core. I wanted to infect her with a slow and painful infection, to reduce her to terror, and then to watch her die. And I also knew that her conscious access to such feelings was a response to my observations about her need and her cruelty. There was a brief moment in which she understood that she associated me with her mother's madness. Indeed, she acknowledged that she could *only establish my real sanity by discovering that I really became infected with a life-threatening illness.* This discovery would indicate that I was not malingering or reclusive, but rather a sane maternal object. But at the very moment when she would discover my maternal sanity, she would have lost me and perhaps killed me. She could almost imagine remorse at my death. And then she retreated to her contempt, insisting that I was delusional, or absurdly fearful of the most minor ailments. At the end of the session, I reiterated my insistence that she not attend session again in this condition. She agreed to comply.

Two weeks later, I canceled her session because of a flu. I struggled not to sink into a paranoid rage that this was indeed the flu that she, personally, had inflicted on me. On the day of her canceled session, I received a rare phone call from her requesting a return call late in the evening. Still assuming her basic human decency, I assumed it must be an emergency to justify a phone call on a day of illness. I stayed awake to return the call. When I was able to reach her, she attempted to keep me on the phone with a lengthy discussion of insurance forms. I was enraged. The following week she became belligerent about my curtness on the phone, complaining that I was an inadequate professional. When I drew her attention to the fact that she knew I was ill that day, she expressed the view that my illness was not really real, or really severe enough to justify a day off. She acknowledged that she had purposely called me when I was sick. Indeed, she had entertained the fantasy that she had actually given me this cold by coming sick to session. This statement was cold and flat, and contained no guilt. I observed that she must have wanted to force her mother to come out and provide for her, and that if mother would not come out, Donna would go in and torment her.

Subsequently, she developed an ambiguous mild cough, which placed me in a double bind. It was as if the cough were taunting me: it was serious enough to make me anxious, and mild enough to subvert the limits I had established. Certainly, I would seem quite psychotic to make a fuss about it; to forbid her to come with it would virtually mean terminating. Perhaps that was its meaning. The cough disappeared and reappeared, always eluding accountability and analysis. Even as she coughed, she made impossible and contradictory demands for special treatment arrangements: late hours, changing hours, special billing, and so on. With these escalating demands, which I must inevitably fail to meet, she seemed to be bartering for my life: mother me or I'll kill you. All the while, she knew herself much as she knew her uncle: kind and strong, without need and without cruelty.

And even as she coughed, we began to discover another aspect of her uncle. He was authoritarian, possessive, and tyrannical, a man who had solicited his sister's dependency, a man who engaged in the torment of his sister by inviting Donna to treat her own mother with sadism and contempt. He had driven his sister ever further into reclusive madness, much as Donna drove me and her lover further into reclusive dread as a defense against Donna's onslaughts. And in the same period of analysis, Donna pursued contact with her mother, and discovered in her mother an untapped nurturant capacity. These discoveries disorganized her entire relational matrix; I wondered if she would have the strength to sustain herself in this disorganization. There were so many times when our dialogue seemed at the brink of a breakthrough. But our words never reached into the encounter occurring between our bodies. She coughed and expelled her toxicity, she coughed and taunted me with the prospect of my death. I felt strangely imprisoned with her in my struggle for survival. While my mind held her in analytic understanding, my body communicated to her that her body was bad and that her rage and her hunger were going to be my destruction.

In relation to her sadistic self, I was in a state of terror and hatred. But in relation to her abandoned infant self, I was haunted by bestial guilt. It was true, what I observed about her infantile sadistic self. But what is also true is that she was carrying the real weight of her analyst's life, of her analyst's death. She was carrying my real and relentless accusation. Her "resistance to the awareness of the transference" (Gill, 1982) was the more tenacious because I held her responsible for

destroying the analyst's (presumably) fragile sense of self . . .
in these circumstances, some analysands will hear any
interpretive intervention as a condemnation, specifically, a
condemnation borne of the analyst's fragility and sense of
having been damaged [Greenberg, 1999, p. 144].

If she heard this condemnation, she heard me accurately. I
could not manage the lonely prospect of my own annihilation. I
made her carry it. And in this I betrayed her. I should have transferred her to a healthy analyst whom she could not destroy with
her bodily toxins. But I could not admit that I could be destroyed.
Each time I neared my own dread, my grandiosity located endless
pathways away from it. These pathways erected fissures of the
mind, creating a disjunction of remembering and forgetting. *I for-*
*got that I could no longer empathize with a patient who might have*
*infected me with death. I forgot the murderous dread that can attend the*
*awakening of an annihilated infant. I forgot that an analyst cannot require*
*such an infant to meet the analyst's dread with depressive integration, repa-*
*ration, and concern. I forgot that such an infant needs an analyst who will*
*not die of the patient's toxicity. I forgot that I could not make such a*
*promise. Above all, I forgot that honor is eventually forfeited in the immi-*
*nence of extinction. I sometimes think that I forgot almost everything I*
*knew, because to remember would have been a surrender to mortality. I*
*could not surrender.*

In such an analytic context, her infant self could only awaken
and then return to damnation. Our analysis consolidated her
infantile experience of badness. Her sadism and her hunger were
reevacuated into silence. She terminated analysis in a schizoid
compromise. Citing a series of concrete impediments (fees, hours,
insurance limitations), she indicated that continued sessions were
not feasible. She did not, would not, attribute her termination to
our mutual destructiveness.

She seemed to simply enter a dead zone. Now I remember her
as I last saw her: a still snapshot, a vacuity, an analytic casualty no
longer in search of her own interior. She would not seek analysis
again. Analysts were mad as mother was mad. Babies were bad and
their bodies were bad. As her analyst, as a healer, I survived her

destruction, but I feel ethically abased. What if I had transferred her? I would have been haunted by guilt for precipitiously abandoning her without attempting to work it through. And perhaps her infant self would have met this abandonment with another schizoid compromise. I still cannot imagine a path that would have enabled us both to stay alive: me in my body, and her in her mind. I have only my guilt to occupy the space where our living relation should have been.

I survived. But I have never said goodbye. I am well now. For many years, my body is intact, and my guilt is interminable. I know myself as her perpetrator. I barely remember her sadistic self, which required analytic containment. The events, the "facts," exist in my notes. I remember only her emergent infant self, my professional responsibility, my own failure and transgressions. My guilt occludes the historical truth of her cruelty. Like most survivors, I want death for having wanted life. I re-imagine those early days, and find myself embracing a "noble" death. I do not banish her from my office at that moment when she reveals her walking pneumonia. I impale myself on her toxicity, risk infection. In this vision, I reverse the bestial core of my own survival. In the death of my self, I restore my self: I repossess my own ethical subjectivity.

## CONCLUSION

In the absence of the reparative death, survivors live in an abortive relation to reparative hunger. Those who retain bestial guilt and bestial memory survive in masochism, and tend toward revictimization. In this masochism, the survivor sustains the condition of existential mindfulness, in which the ethical contradictions of survival cannot be dissociated or foreclosed. She cannot forget that mankind "is set apart while being a part; he is homeless, yet chained to the home he shares with all creatures. . . . He is never free from the dichotomy of his existence: he cannot rid himself of his mind, even if he would want to; he cannot rid himself of his body as long as he is alive—and his body makes him want to be alive" (Fromm, 1964, p. 253).

And while she turns accusation and remembrance against the self, so she retains an image of goodness. She exists in a nascent depressive subjectivity, in the potentiality of object-related concern and hatred.

This potentiality resides in the predicament of masochism. For the masochistic survivor has often found that her own bestial gesture was met by the perpetrator's deadness, by his satisfaction and contempt. In such a context, an immoral act continues to be registered as immoral: the perpetrator's very contempt consolidates the victim's guilt and sense of otherness. As long as the survivor retains a sense of agency and remorse, some autonomous fragment of the survivor continues to live in reparative longing. And if she has had some opportunity to offer tenderness to other victims in their own abasement, she will retain the memory and the inspiration of goodness (see Todorov, 1996).

But for those like Donna for whom loss, guilt, and despair are void, survival is transmuted into the manic defense of cruelty and contempt (see Segal, 1964). Here, "the death fear of the ego is lessened by the killing, the sacrifice of the other; through the death of the other, one buys oneself free from the penalty of dying, of being killed" (Rank, 1936, p. 130). Such survivors exist in the condition of forgetfulness; they will neither remember their own transgression, nor will they register an accusation against their own oppressor. In such cruelty and forgetfulness, the existential problem of survival is foreclosed, and all conflict is silenced. The ethics of the mind and the survival of the body no longer live in an impossible, but authentic antagonism. This survivor does not want death for wanting life; she wants another's moral abasement.

If the good, masochistic survivor locates her nascent goodness in the interpersonal conditions of her trauma, so the cruel survivor likewise locates the origins of her cruelty. When the trauma victim is welcomed into the perpetrator's approving embrace *after* the victim's moral transgression, if her own torture ceases *after* her bestial gesture, if she has had no cohorts with whom to make a reparative gesture, and if this annihilation occurred in childhood before the depressive self was consolidated, guilt may be permanently eradicated. This is not only due to identification with the aggressor, and the states of terror, pain, confusion described so eloquently in the work of Lifton (1961), Shatan (1977), Lifton and Markhusen (1990), and Herman (1992). It is due, as Laub and Auerhahn (1989) might suggest, to the inventing of an empathic other in the perpetrator, who is the victim's only human link, the only mirroring object. In my view, this establishes a structure in which the victim's need to make a reparative gesture has been deprived of all but one object: the perpetrator. And the perpetrator appears to be loved and made whole again by the survivor's moral transgression. Where there was either schizoid deadness or murderous chaos within the perpetrator, there is now warmth, an apparently benign communion with the victim. The perpetrator is manifestly restored to "sanity" by the victim's inhuman act. Now survival, ethical concern, reparative longings, and agency suddenly appear coextensive, where they have been in existential conflict: the victim can be "good" and nonetheless take manic flight from the memory of annihilation and despair. Reparative and manic defenses collapse into one another in a labyrinth of defensive sadism. One "loves" through the restoration of one's perpetrator; one "loves" through the denial of pain and of one's own history; one "loves" through the torture of another. In a modified sense, this dynamism is operative in Donna's family system: she brings her depressed uncle to life by tormenting the mother, even as she consolidates her attachment to him as her only available object. Such processes may underlie what Lifton (1986) describes as the "healing–killing paradox" of warfare and genocidal culture, wherein one is encouraged to kill in order to "heal" one's own damaged or endangered community. Once immersed in the healing–killing paradox, one experiences no moral transgression; one need not want death for wanting life. One need only inflict death. And so, the reproduction of evil locates its endgame.

# CHAPTER 6

# THE DEPRAVITIES OF THE NONHUMAN SELF: GREED, MURDER, PERSECUTION

I HAD JUST RETURNED FROM MY SUMMER VACATION. My office was cool and still and expectant, the way an analytic room is when it has long been empty of stories. Claire and I took our seats. She studied each object in its place. Then she began to speak. Over the next few sessions, I listened for the man who was missing from her stories. Prior to my vacation, he had consumed her. Where he was present, now he was absent. As I listened, the room's tranquility filled with dim perception. I sensed, rather than knew, that he was gone. First, gone; then, dead; then, finally: murdered. Murdered by my patient, during my vacation. And she had told me nothing.

As surely as I sensed his murder, just as surely did my conviction vanish. I looked again, and there she was: articulate, intelligent, petite, feminine. She was a graduate student, a competent professional, a child of middle class suburbia. She was a woman in search of an autonomous self, a girl who collapsed into nothingness in relation to a man. With a man, she could barely speak and assert herself on her own behalf. Not with her lover. Not with her father. With a man, she experienced her own fate as accidental. To Claire, man was a saint and man was a devil; she could only receive him.

As I moved closer to the interior of this self-abnegation, I had been struck by some intractable chaos, some erotic link to self-destruction. In the past, she had been beaten by boyfriends. After work, marijuana use rendered her docile, conciliatory; it filled her hollows, and consigned her anger to oblivion. Now she had become enmeshed with the marijuana "connection" who had taunted and threatened her, stashing heroin and cocaine in her apartment. He had been demanding that she collude in its sale, occupying her home, refusing to leave it. With him, she had been mute, impotent, diminished, a supplicant defined by the man, and violated by his definition. About him, she had been urgent, terrified, loquacious. For two months prior to my vacation, not a session had passed without stories of her fear, and of her impotent assertions. Not a session had passed without our examination of solutions, of her drug use, of her unwitting solicitation of his trespass, and of her unwitting expectation of her own defeat. It began to seem that the solution was simple: were she to vacate the apartment, ceding it to him, he would passively relinquish his hold over her. I sensed that he would not stalk her. But what seemed simple to me appeared to her as an impossibility. On the topic of her apartment she was strangely intractable: she could not, would not, leave it to his possession. It was *hers*. It was in this impasse that I left her, prior to my vacation.

Now, upon my return from vacation, there was neither complaint, nor fear, nor hate, nor triumph. There was not any form of continuity. He had simply fallen away into silence. I wanted to ask about him. Questions seemed lethal and knowledge seemed toxic. It was this very toxicity that aroused my suspicion. But then I thought: *passive girls don't kill.* Just as my intuition began to lose itself in her masochism, she told me. She wanted to bring me her authentic self, and that self was lived out in the night of the murder.

During my absence, the "connection" had continued in his drug trafficking, in his bold refusal to leave her home. He slept in a separate room. There was no sex, and there was no rape. Sometimes, she imagined rape as imminent. But he was essentially stuporous, indifferent, and immovable, a sleeping bully one dare not awaken. She was violated by the possibility of his sexual menace, and she was violated by his lack of erotic recognition. But she was violated most by his possession of her own apartment, an apartment she would not leave. And so, she planned it. She waited until night fell. He was asleep. She injected him with an overdose of heroin, and waited for the cessation of his breathing. He would not die, and his death was imperative. She took a pillow and smothered him. His limbs fell still. Disposing of the drugs in the apartment, but not the drugs on his body, she passed the night in her bedroom. His corpse lay in the other room. In the morning she "discovered" his body and contacted the police. There were tracks on his arms, drugs in his bloodstream. She was intelligent, White, feminine, middle class, professional. The "connection" was solitary, Hispanic, transient, a tatooed, foul-smelling, gold-chained "piece of scum." According to the police, there was no murder. They envisioned her as a victimized good-girl; they envisioned him as dying from a self-inflicted overdose.

She went to his funeral. In the weeks afterward, she went to work, socialized, and got stoned. Life was dim and unreal and infused with expectancy and waiting. Her own limbs felt like wood blocks, clumsy, disjointed, set loose from her human frame. This self was a "machine." "It" moved as if through several passages of glass: severed and encapsulated, insensate to everything but cold. Only in the apartment did "it" feel real and whole. In the apartment there was a sense of blissful remoteness from all human transaction. This bliss was not human, but a merger of a thing among things: it was as if ocean and earth had fused after repelling mankind's depredations. In this way, the apartment and Claire constituted an inorganic landscape. Void of human trespass, the apartment was renewed in its tranquility. In this state she was secret. As a therapist, as a human, I could not meet this thing-self of primordial bliss that emerged in the solitude of things. Instead I met the "machine." It was the machine that had arrived in session after my vacation. It was the machine who committed the murder and who told me about the blissful experience in the apartment.

I asked her why she had killed him after months of timidity, deference, and capitulation. I asked why she did not leave her apartment, move out, seek help, intervention. She did not speak of rage, of shame, or of justice, nor of protecting or avenging an abused feminine self. She could not answer in any terms that would allow us to retain a human link. She answered only in the language of things: "*I had to kill him for the apartment.*"

Now I recalled that my first clue to the murder was in the context of things and their human violation. I did not find my first clue in her silence about the "connection." I found it in my office, just prior to our arrival. Then, my office was as her apartment: its empty tranquility was derived from human absence. Later, its violation was derived from the renewal of human presence. I knew this as she made her confession. And as she made her confession, her body shifted and grew before me, until she attained a certain hard muscular volatility. Her wooden limbs knit and found the sudden grace of violence. Her voice, pitched low, became a taunt, a fist, an embodied ultimatum, and I knew its implication: "I have murdered for the apartment, I will stay in the apartment. Do not become another human impediment."

In the sessions after her confession, I was only referred to as the "witness": where I had possessed a name, I possessed it no longer. I too existed at the threshold of thingness. I felt deprived of speech, even with those agency administrators and lawyers with whom I had discussed her confession. By day, I worked. But time was out of joint; it had no defined surfaces. My dreams were devoid of all human character: there were beasts and floods and storms in a landscape bereft of all humanity. In waking fantasy, I anticipated myself as a murdered corpse, inert and thing-discarded. I saw my body lying in dim streets, body parts in black body bags, chalk on the sidewalk. Unidentified and unidentifiable. Alive, I had knowledge of a murder that did not exist. I was an anonymous thing-container for an event that had eluded human accountability because *it was not human.* His life and my life, his corpse and my corpse, his murder and my witnessing: we were mere keys to the lock on her interiority. And it was precisely this key, this irreducible thingness, that would unlock the door to her traumatic memory.

## GREED'S ALCHEMY:
## ANNIHILATION AND THING-POSSESSION

The "connection" was the apartment's usurper. Claire murdered him for its possession. Her fear and her abjection: these were not the essential object of *his* desire. His death and her vengeance: these were not the true object of *her* desire. For this couple, the dynamism of sadomasochism was the surface for a more inexplicable engagement. It was the humanized text for a nonhuman hunger. Her subjection and his corpse were incidental to their purpose, mere props in the pursuit of thing possession. Their passions were not for one another; their lusts were not filled in each other's torment. No: their sin was avarice, their passion was a *greed for the thing in itself*. The wealth to be accrued from the selling of illegal drugs, the "turf" to be gained through the sole possession of the apartment: these *things* were their beloved. Human destruction was simply the means to a covetous end.

So it has been throughout human history, that violence is inspired by the hunger for thing-possession. Greed surpasses all moral parameters. In the "search for a meal in the midst of a banquet" (Barton, 1993), mankind seems impelled toward infinite aggression and perversity. Unsated and insatiable, craven in his acquisitive desire, mankind eradicates all human impediments to possession. Money, land, material power: for these, wars are fought, slaves are taken, individuals and entire cultures are exploited, annihilated, and oppressed. In evil's deformation of ethics, the human and the nonhuman seem linked in a reversal: that which is human is reduced to an it, and that which is an *it* is rendered sacred. Greed's victim is filled with every dimension of human suffering. And yet he is it-defined: envisioned by the perpetrator as devoid of all the enlightened shadows of human subjectivity. This is the contradictory status of greed's victim: to be seen as a shallow thing, emptied of all subjectivity, and yet to be used as a full container for human suffering. To define the victim as an "it" while using the victim as pain's container: this is a "magical remedy" that permits the perpetrator to injure and to deny the victim's injury (also see

Ogden, 1989). It allows him to "expunge from history the harm that was done. History is rewritten and the need for guilt is thereby obviated" (Ogden, 1989, p. 23). Even in death, greed's victim is defined by the thingness of corpses. What was a living interior is now inert, thing-discarded. A corpse functions as the repository for all that reviled filth that exists at the margins of human existence: the fecal, the decay of all creatures. And through this most magical of remedies, that filth, that thing, disappears into a grave. And the coveted object of greed remains suffused with that golden light which should inhere in human life.

As the novelist Unsworth (1992) suggests, African-American slavery was the exemplar of this lunatic exchange:

> The tall negro . . . was purchased finally for six brass kettles, two cabers of cowries, four silver-laced cocked hats, twenty-five looking glasses and an anker of brandy, with a bonus of six folding knives and a plumed hat [p. 210].

For pedestrian implements, for the glint of brass and silver and glass, for the glitter of beads and the plumage of hats, an African is kidnapped and sold to a slave ship. To breed new slaves, to produce limitless free labor for the generation of a white master's wealth, African women are packed into the slave hold. As things, they possessed nothing: not their bodies, nor their lives, nor the lives of their children; not even the rough boards upon which they slept. Their condition of humanity was, as Soyinka (1999) suggests, one of denial:

> "You can get up to a hundred in there, if you stow
> em spoon-fashion, arse by tit"
> "Bigob, a hundred black fannies," Billy said [p. 174].

Suffocating in the hold, dehumanized by rape and by filth and stench and chains, severed from love, forbidden all speech, craving the food that their masters dispense, a human victim becomes a thing (Owens, 1953; Genovese, 1972; Fox-Genovese, 1988). Her body, and the bodies of her beloved, become mere planks in the church of her abductor:

Deep in the festering hold thy father lies,
of his bones New England pews are made,
those are altar lights that were his eyes
[Robert Hayden, "Middle Passage," in Chapman, 1968).

And because the perpetrator exalts the thing, even as the
human slave is reduced to an it, there is no mutual recognition of
the slave's subjective history. Historical records of business transactions concerned only the white men; the slave was "but an object
coloring the circumstances" (Troutt, 1998, p. 2). It is precisely the
invisible thingness of the slaves' condition that "coerces and
induces (the) forgetfulness" of them in subsequent American law
(Troutt, 1998, p. 2). We hear that occlusion of memory and justice
in Douglass's (1845) slave narrative:

"No matter how innocent a slave might be—it availed him
nothing . . . to be accused was to be convicted, and to be
convicted was to be punished; the one always following the
other with immutable certainty. To escape punishment was
to escape accusation, and few slaves had the fortune to do
either . . . (the overseer) was cruel enough to inflict the
severest punishment, artful enough to descend to the lowest
trickery, and obdurate enough to be insensible to the voice
of a reproving conscience. . . . He spoke but to command
and commanded but to be obeyed; he dealt sparingly with
his words and bountifully with his whip" [p. 46].

On the slave ship, (as on the plantation), the despair of slaves
was met only by slaves: by those human others who have been
defined as utilitarian objects, as the mere implements of wealth.
These slaves, suffering their bondage, are stripped of human history. Their pain is not witnessed by those whom history has
located as human: the master class. They become the "unthinkable
thing-in-itself" (Ogden, 1997, p. 34). Unheard by "human" ear,
unwitnessed by "human" eye, the slaves' anguish resounds in the
night and in the sea, until the abduction of slaves seems registered
in the seascape itself:

But when the ship met the deep sea swell, the rhythm of her movement changed and the people in the cramped and fetid darkness of the hold, understanding that they had lost all hope of returning to their homes, set up a great cry of desolation and despair that carried over the water to other ships in the road and the slaves in the holds of the ships heard it and answered with wild shouts and screams, so that . . . there was a period when the night resounded with the echoes of lamentation [Unsworth, 1992, p. 304].

In Unsworth's evocative fiction, *Sacred Hunger*, the seascape severs slaves from home and swallows up their dead. And yet, even as the slave is defeated by the sea, so Unsworth's seascape appears as both advocate and witness: it provides the slaves' bondage with an eternal, historic inscription. Their truth has resounded in its waters: its night tides are the same night tides that touch us now, four hundred years later. One has the sense that the slaves' cries have found an infinite echo on the ocean's surface, even as the slaves' skeletons are held within its depth. And so the slave, reduced to a thing, seems to be witnessed by the thing: not by human rescue and compassion, but by the ocean's testimonial to its dead. Tracing the route of the Atlantic slave trade, the Nigerian essayist Soyinka (1999) evokes this testimonial:

of all the landmarks of slavery I had ever traversed, none, not even the grim tunnels of Goree or Cape Coast, worn smooth by the yet echoing slaps of feet on the passage into hell, could match the eerie evocation of the walk toward Embarkation Point . . . we . . . passed over flagstones worn smooth by the boots of slave owners and the bare feet of slaves. . . . No experience however could match the long walk through clumps of mangrove and palms, with clutches of huts and palm frond encased compounds in pristine preservation, along the only safe path through treacherous marine ponds and mangrove swamps. As if by common consent, we breathed gently, as if we feared to disturb a somnolent air that had lain on the earth, seem-

ingly undisturbed for centuries . . . and so, all the way to
the embarkation point, and the place of no return. . . .
There was only a quiescent residuum of history as palpa-
ble reality, as truth [pp. 65–68].

In the pathways worn smooth, in the stagnance of the air, there
is the "yet echoing slap" of slave feet. The slave, reduced to an "it,"
voiceless in human discourse, is coerced in his body as a mere
stone among stones. But if he is voiceless in human discourse, he
is not so in nonhuman discourse: the stone pathway memorializes
his dread. The slave's history waits, until a human witness listens to
the language of the earth.

## THINGNESS AND THE BESTIAL GESTURE OF SURVIVAL

The slap of feet becomes the slave's only monologue of memory.
As a stone among stones the slave is annihilated and forgotten; as
a stone among stones, we find the possibility of his remembrance.
This paradox foreshadows the slave's bestial gesture of survival. For,
in annihilation's abasement, the slave's internal relation to his own
thingness must become divided. He is forced to embrace that very
thingness that has oppressed him. That thing-reduction which has
been the source of his pain now becomes his only escape into
invisibility. The victim discovers that he can numb his terror and
leave his body by hypnotically fusing with environmental things.
Like the rape victim focusing on the wallpaper, becoming that
wallpaper, and viewing her body from above (Herman, 1992), the
slave may take flight by merging with things.

And if thingness seduces with its nullification of pain, so it may
provide an escape from the personalized sadisms of the perpetrator. Where once the slave "merely" suffered the anonymous instru-
mental cruelties of abduction, now, on the plantation, she
encounters whole new realms of torture. What began as a malign
oblivion to the slave's human rights became a hate for, and fear of,
the slave. The master class evolved persecutory anxiety regarding

rebellion, violence, and the rape of white women. They controlled their slaves and took vengeance on them, through an extraordinary inventory of bodily tortures (see Genovese, 1976; Fox-Genovese, 1988). In what slim agentic margin remained to the slave, she often contrived to conceal her human existence and to make herself "thing-invisible." Thus, the good "house nigger" tried to make herself indistinguishable from the appearance of food and the removal of china. In this, she hopes to conceal her human vaginal aperture and avoid the master's rape and the mistress's beating. Through this merger with the thing, she strives to leave the perpetrator alone without an object of torment: "In a world where one was alone there could be no victims, and so there could be no cruelty" (Barton, 1993, p. 56). And so, to paraphrase Soyinka (1999), the oppressed may greet the nonhuman self, "hailing its birth in the same breath" as they "elegantly weave its shroud."

## IMMORTALITY AND POSSESSION: THE ALCHEMY OF GREED

How shall we understand that strange alchemy of greed which exchanges the sacred for the profane? What urgency drives mankind's "sacred hunger" (Unsworth, 1992), impelling him to reduce human life to base metal, while conferring life's numinosity onto the base metal of things? I propose that it is the paranoid-schizoid desire for immortality that drives greed's violence. And through paranoid-schizoid splitting and projective identification, greed's discarded human victim becomes the repository for all earthly mortality (see Riviere, 1964, on greed, splitting, and projective identification). Ominous as the signifer of suffering and mortality, the victim must now be killed, so that human suffering will not cast its shadow over the tyrant's omnipotence. Through the continual renewal of violence, acquisitors deny that:

> Their grave is their eternal home,
> the dwelling place for all generations
> of those once famous on the earth
> [Psalm 49, verses 6–11].

How odd that base things should seem to promise immortality. What a strange notion this is. And yet, we must postulate such a link with thing-possession, if we are to excavate the primordial violence of greed. Indeed, Shakespeare, that great observer of mankind, seems to propose such a link in *Macbeth*. For *Macbeth* may be read as a testimonial to mankind's archaic imagining that thing-possession will release him from his "mortal coil." Thus, Lady Macbeth exhorts her God to

> fill me, from the crown to the toe, top-full
> Of direst cruelty!
> make thick my blood
> Stop up th'access and passage to
> remorse [Lady Macbeth, *Macbeth,* act I, scene 5].

so that the Macbeths can kill the king and steal the king's crown for Macbeth's head. Through the king's murder, she and Macbeth will acquire all that the rightful king has possessed: power, land, wealth. Exultant in the promise of possession, it is as if Lady Macbeth envisions herself, staring out at her kingdom's vistas, crying: this earth, this sky, this sea, *these are mine.* Bejeweled, glowing with rare gold and infinite power, the crown seems to signify ownership of that "massive transcendance of creation" (Becker, 1973), "which the eye never has enough of seeing/Nor the ear enough of hearing" (Ecclesiastes 1:2–8). Through immoral acts, the crown's thief will attain nature's immortal power, and find release from his mortal form. Macbeth must "screw his courage to the sticking-place" so that mere manhood can become a royal, godlike dominion. He has simply to leap across the abyss of violence to find himself in a realm beyond extinction, and beyond human conscience.

And so, for the crown's possession, he kills the king; in its possession he imagines himself a king who cannot be killed. Failing to apprehend the paradox of this possession, he heeds only the prophecy of his omnipotence: once in possession of the crown, it is foretold that Macbeth cannot be killed by any man of woman born. It is here that Shakespeare speaks to the fantastic equation of immortality and thing-possession.

And it is here that he speaks of greed's tragic implications: like the ancient Romans (see Barton, 1993), Macbeth's wanting only grows through its gratification, becoming cancerous in its renewed desire, perverse in its pleasure, until pleasure itself threatens to become a torment. He has gained the crown, and yet, his thirst for immortality remains unslaked. There is an "exhaustion of the possible [which] created a desire for the ultimate and the impossible . . . the tyrant, the man most capable of indulging his wishes, was the man most afflicted by lunatic desire" (Barton, 1993, pp. 53–54).

Women and children are slaughtered in the excess of his hunger. Mortality and grief and pain reside in the bodies of his subjects, while Macbeth's arrogant claim to immortality grows with every violent assertion of his crown. But Shakespeare teaches us that immortality belongs to nature. If Macbeth has sequestered himself in prophesies and illusions, still he cannot elude death. The crown is his, but it is a circle of base metal, void of all magic, powerless to secure him from bodily frailty. He wears it. Lady Macbeth's suicide briefly stirs him. In this morbid stillness, he perceives the futility of all he has desired, the talismanic emptiness of his crown:

> To-morrow, and tomorrow, and to-morrow,
> Creeps in this petty pace from day to day,
> To the last syllable of recorded time;
> And all our yesterdays have lighted fools
> The way to dusty death. Out, out, brief candle!
> Life's but a walking shadow; a poor player,
> That struts and frets his hour upon the stage,
> And then is heard no more: it is a tale
> Told by an idiot, full of sound and fury,
> Signifying nothing [*Macbeth,* act 5, scene 5].

But despair is unbearable, as truth is unbearable; Macbeth takes flight through the "lavish waste of the spoils of war, the wealth that rages to its ruin" (Petronius in *Satyricon* as quoted in Barton, 1993, p. 55). Nonetheless, justice pursues him, and he encounters the confines of his own corporeal being. He encounters Macduff, former friend turned figure of vengeance, whose family Macbeth has slaughtered. Macduff, a man not of woman born, but one who "was from his mother's womb/Untimely ripp'd" (Macduff, act 5, scene 5), was delivered into the world as his mother died in childbirth. Now, newly aggrieved by loss, Macduff is unable to forget that death terminates all human life. It is Macduff's sword that pierces the delusional link between greed and immortality. Still possessed of his crown, Macbeth dies on Macduff's just sword, startled in his mortality, unrepentant, and naked in his dread.

## IMMORTALITY AND THE NONHUMAN SELF

The connection's murder, the structure of slavery, and the portrayal of *Macbeth*, although vastly different in some respects, are nonetheless common in their basic unconscious assumption that acquiring the thing means *becoming* the thing and, *in that becoming, a man may possess immortality*. If the threat of annihilation reduces the body to abjection and to that "determinism and boundedness . . . [which is] a shadow on the person's inner freedom" (Becker, 1973, p. 42), then it seems inevitable that mankind seeks to escape his human form. What is more natural than to flee one's human embodiment in search of another form, a form defined by its existence outside of death? And, "what is more natural to banish one's fears than to live on delegated powers?" (Becker, 1973, p. 23). To fuse with immortality by escaping one's human form, one must have recourse to the inorganic world, where "death shall have no dominion" (Thomas, 1952). In a sufficiency of possession, in a magical fusion with the inorganic aspect of things, mankind can void his human form and merge with the infinitude of the natural world.

While elements of omnipotent fusion can be gained in narcissistic forms of human relatedness (Bach, 1994), ultimately all human interchange is redolent with the bodily imminence of death. By contrast, inorganic things are defined by a singular and enviable aspect: *they cannot die*. Although the inanimate can be destroyed by external forces, they are insensate and unaffected by an internal process of dying. And if inanimate objects promise a reprieve from the anticipation of death, the "massive transcendance of creation" promises infinitude. Even as we die, behold: a world thrilling with eternal life.

## Searles and the Nonhuman Self

Perhaps the capacity for merger with the inorganicity and immortality of things derives from the nonhuman area of self described by Searles (1960). Searles provides an evocative sense of a moment in development in which one is undifferentiated, not merely from the human other, but from the nonhuman environment. This stratum of the self is ungendered. For Searles, when human environmental contact is barren, cruel, or depriving, developmental differentiation from the nonhuman may fail to occur. As a result, subsequent experiences of dread, instability, and helplessness result in a regressive craving for, and merger with, the nonhuman. Any loss of nonhuman supports is akin to a *mutilation of the body*, as if one were dismembered. In such a regression, the annihilation of the human self is escaped through a merger with the enduring constancy of *things*, and with the associated resurrection of the nonhuman self. The loss of human connection is death's *penultimate* moment. It is the loss of thing attachments, *not the loss of human attachments*, that represents the ultimate and final psychic death. In excavating his patients' terror and disorganization at being severed from their nonhuman environment, Searles recognizes another world within the human world. He finds retreats within retreats, all aimed at eluding extinction. When annihilation anxiety threatens, his patients seek a preserving link with the beneficence of nonhuman stasis. When this link collapses, there is no end to dying. All of the self dies, every fragment, every piece.

In his unique analysis, Searles grasps the urgency of the human-thing relation without eviscerating this relation of its most vital attribute: inorganicity. He recognizes the benign inertness of things, their constancy, their autonomy from human bonds. And while he does not address the role of evil in the human-thing relation, his analysis is suggestive. Perhaps the murderer's human self is the fragile survivor of annihilation. If he has survived, like Claire, through a merger with inviolable things, then a perpetual lust for thing-merger operates within him as his singular barrier to extinction. If his psychic death comes, not to his human form, but to his *nonhuman self in relation to his nonhuman objects*, then all human impediments to thing-possession must, and can be, eliminated.

Such a vision resonates with Fromm's (1964) necrophilous character, whose violence is "driven by the desire to transform the organic into the inorganic . . . all living processes, feelings and thoughts are transformed into things . . . the necrophilous person can relate to an object . . . only if he possesses it; hence a threat to his possession is a threat to himself . . . if he loses possession, he loses contact with the world" (p. 41). It resonates as well with Freud's (1920) vision of the human organism as driven by a "demonic" need to return to an inorganic state, to those "inanimate things [which] existed before living ones" (Freud, 1920, p. 38).

## Splitting, Projective Identification, and the Cruelties of the Nonhuman Self

Inevitably, human-to-human encounters threaten the survivor with the memory of his own annihilation. In such moments, the greed of the nonhuman self escalates in proportion to the resurgence of dread. The nonhuman self is akin to that psychotic area of the self described by P. Williams (1998) (note: in this quote the use of the word *object* may be confusing. It does not connote the inorganic thing, but rather, it is the term used by neo-Kleinians for the human other):

> This malformed psychic organism was incapable of relating to any object . . . [it had] an object-alien discourse . . . presymbolic, asymptotic, at once idealizing, omniscient and lethally paranoid . . . its objective seems to be to generate massive distraction from genuine objects. The psychotic personality did not belong to, and was repelled by, the world of objects [Williams, 1998, pp. 462–463].

Repelled by human others, suffused with the urgent hunger for immortal life—now the nonhuman self discovers the need to locate human dread outside the self in a "bad" and dispensable human Other. When we speak of fusion with the immortal object, when we speak of dread's displacement into another who must then be exterminated as the repository of our dread, we are speaking of a self located in the paranoid–schizoid modality (see e.g., Klein, 1946; Segal, 1957; Bion, 1962; Riviere, 1964; Grotstein, 1981; Ogden, 1989; Pye, 1996; Eigen, 1998). Like the autistic–contiguous modality, the paranoid–schizoid modality fears extinction and is mobilized around a refusal of dread; like the autistic–contiguous modality, it cannot locate others as autonomous human *subjects*. But unlike the autistic contiguous mode, survival is not predicated on the reassuring tactile surfaces of things, but on the oral incorporation of goodness into the self.

Unlike the autistic–contiguous modality, here in the paranoid–schizoid modality, there are rudimentary visions of self and other. Self and other are interrelated through either fusion/incorporation or attack/expulsion. In the paranoid–schizoid universe, visions of the self and other cannot embrace any possibility of subject-to-subject dialogue, nor can they sustain shadows of ambiguity. Everything is categorized as either good (facilitating of life) or bad (attacking, destroying, ending in starvation and death). The self and the object world are a sphere of infernal chaos and part objects; this world exalts in omnipotent powers, only to collapse before imminent destruction. The paranoid–schizoid self is without an interpreting subject, and without a continuous personal history. The history of its object relations is rewritten a thousand times a day (Ogden, 1989, 1990) as the self moves urgently between the incorporation of goodness and the expulsion of badness. Here, goodness equals omniscient life. An encounter with badness means a collapse into "endless worlds of deadness" (Bion as referred to by Eigen, 1998, p. 185). Because there are no interim worlds between good and bad, because there are no subtleties in the perception of objects, splitting and projective identification are utilized to segregate badness from goodness. As Ogden (1990) notes, splitting is a boundary-creating mode of thought, not a meaning-generating

process. The paranoid–schizoid modality operates through concrete symbolic equation, that is, thought is concrete and does not
recognize symbols as symbols. Despite greedy efforts to incorpo-
rate goodness, the state of internal goodness versus external badness never reaches equilibrium. Bad stuff is always threatening
invasion, and good stuff is forever withdrawing. Greed is never
sated, and projective identification must be constantly renegotiated
to keep disintegration at bay. Bad stuff must be continually ejected
outward into an external container, and this container must then
be attacked to insure that badness does not take its revenge on the
self. In this continuous flux, and in the absence of a historical subject, there is no continuum of time. This modality is characterized
by a kind of amnesia about the past in which others are used as
"containers" of all the unmetabolized "bad stuff" in the self. These
part object containers are forgotten, void of subjectivity, fungible,
nonhuman, readily discarded. Even as they are subject to nonsadis-
tic narcissistic usage, they are also subject to the sadism of persecutory anxiety. As the repository of all mortal suffering, these are "bad"
objects, which may return to attack and invade the "good" omniscient self.

And so, we begin to comprehend the dynamism of greed. If
someone has survived a past annihilation and anticipates another;
if survival was linked to an embrace of nonhuman invisibility; if he
seeks to liberate himself from all future death through the incorporation of the nonhuman, then his greed for possession signifies
a desire to *become* as immortal as nature. And if he lives in the
paranoid–schizoid modality of splitting and projective identification, then his covetousness requires a sacrificial human life. This
sacrificial human life (the victim, the slave) functions as the fungible "it" devoid of an interior *and also* as the repository of dread.
Human extinction must reside exclusively in the Other, so that the
self has sole access to the source of infinitude. Such splitting and
projective identification allow the acquisitor to pursue pure nonhuman fusion with immortality. And the human history of the
oppressed must be lost because the oppressed is not a subject, but
a thing. And it must be lost *because the paranoid–schizoid oppressor is
not a true subject living in a continuum of time.* For perpetrator, and for

survivor, there is neither past nor future, but simply a chaotic *now*: memory does not exist. This process is as tragic as it is depraved: greed is never sated, for immortality can never acrue to human life.

## CLAIRE'S MEMORY: THE THINGNESS OF CORPSES AND THE THINGNESS OF SELF

Murderous in her acts, Claire was murdered in her interior. Insofar as she would speak, she would speak through her nonhuman self. Insofar as I seemed human, she would not speak. At its best, our treatment transpired as if we were things among things. In this peculiar conversation, I gradually sensed her inner world. Bodiless, invisible, she would secure herself from human violation. As an "it" she could find benign relation and attachment. Sun, rain, storms: it was nature that offered evocative resonance to her moods. It was the branches of trees that held her and hid her. In childhood, her furniture was constant, her locked door her protector. She understood the language of things, and became them. From the time she was little, her "real self" spoke exclusively in sign, with trees: her hands were their leaves, their leaves were her hands. Human speech was false, as her human body was false. She always dreamed of electrified wooden boxes, vacant straight-backed chairs, immovable furniture, trees, meadows, winter beaches, lightning, quicksand, snow, rats, wolves, insects. She dreamed repeatedly of a clam, sometimes open, sometimes closed, on an empty beach. There was either intense heat or intense chill. Sometimes she could sense the approach of a human foot. The foot never appeared. In its imminent path, the clam diminished, vulnerable and helpless, resolving "it–self" into something ambiguously vaginal, then disintegrating. Often the clam pulsated on the beach, solitary in tidal pools, unmolested, never assuming a vaginal shape.

Claire's family was damaged by sadism and detachment. The middle child of three siblings, she had an older brother and a younger sister. Her father was obsessed with money and things; he was hard and authoritarian, relentless in his control. He beat Claire's brother. Cold and remote, Claire's mother left her son to the father's beatings. At the age of 10, Claire witnessed her father manually penetrating her sister's vagina. She knew to tell no one. The incest lasted for several years. She and her sister never spoke of it. Claire was ignored and unmolested, neglected but invisible. Unlike her sister, Claire was used for servile functions: for the making of beds and the washing of dishes. She was not raped or beaten, but neither was she seen. Claire was relieved that she was exempt from abuse, but she was nonetheless envious of the violation. She imagined her siblings to be both humanized and destroyed by the father's cruelties. In some sense, she felt that her siblings had been entered into existence, while Claire did not exist. She was *neither the object nor the subject of desire*.

Eclipsed in her humanity, Claire was concealed in an inorganic landscape; there, she was comforted and known only as a thing among things. She was desirous of the human and repelled by human nature. When another child reached out to take or destroy a favorite object, she pushed the child down the stairs. Once, when her mother had forbidden her hoarding and had threatened to intrude into her room in order to throw away certain items, Claire intentionally scalded her mother in the kitchen and dropped heavy objects on her mother's feet, thereby breaking her toes. About this incident Claire felt nothing: she exacted punishment for her mother's abandonment and also insured that her mother, now crippled, would be unable to trespass into the sanctuary of Claire's room, which her mother never again tried to "clean." This room became a chaotic repository of the things in Claire's possession. She began to manipulate her peers so that she was able to steal their money, clothes, and jewelry. She stole cash from her father's wallet, thereby incorporating the omniscient core of her father's self, but also wreaking on him the greatest possible vengeance. He too anticipated annihilation without material acquisition. Her greed grew to greater proportions, ever more hungry, ever more violent. In memory of the erasure of her own humanity, in anticipation of beatings, rape, and human abasement, fusion with thingness signified an exalted barrier to human annihilation. And the human bodies whom she violated in pursuit of the thing—these were empty, fungible, readily discarded. Like her father, she was never caught, held culpable, brought to justice, although she was suspected. Neighbors became suspicious of theft, of "accidental" violence perpetrated on their children. But Claire's perpetrator self assumed a docile feminine exterior, in identification with, and mimicry of, her sister's abasement. And before that docile exterior, suspicion inevitably fell away. In this material, I heard the echo of my own disavowal: *passive girls don't kill.*

These memories were not linear in their revelation, but lived and decoded through her relation to our room and to its objects. And some memories were told by the "machine": the mechanical self she evolved to transact the world of human existence. We conversed in enactment, and in a schizoid transference-countertransference matrix in which both analyst and patient were experienced as inanimate objects (see Akhtar, 1999). She did not experience guilt, but she did not wish to kill again. In some remote way, she conveyed knowledge that something was terribly *wrong.* She underwent drug treatment. After a few months, she was hospitalized, and then referred to a psychiatrist. I have not heard from her again. I imagine her murderous like Cain and, like Cain, itinerant and homeless. And though she is homeless, I imagine her in communion with the earth, and with the things of the earth:

> Now, Loneliness forever and the earth again! . . . Heroic friend, blood-brother of Proud Death . . . have we not crossed the stormy seas alone, and known strange lands, and come again to walk the continent of night and listen to the silence of the earth? . . . Come to me, brother, in the watches of the night, come to me in the secret and most silent heart of darkness, come to me as you always came, bringing to me more the old invincible strength, the *death-less hope,* the triumphant joy and confidence that will storm the ramparts of the earth again [Wolfe, 1957, pp. 179–180].

# CHAPTER 7

# FRANKENSTEIN AND HIS MONSTER:
# GRIEF AND THE ESCAPE FROM GRIEF

✺

IN DEFIANCE OF NATURE, AND IN PURSUIT OF HIS OWN WILL, Frankenstein strives to master the life force. He animates the dead, only to be repelled by the creature he has awakened. In Mary Shelley's classic novel, Frankenstein cannot encounter his creation through love and compassion, but rather, abandons his creature at the moment of its "birth." Innocent, hungering for love and interminably reviled, the Creature undergoes what Sullivan (1953) calls the "malevolent transformation." The benign Creature becomes a Monster who seeks his maker through the incremental slaughter of all those whom Frankenstein loves. As death itself pursues him, Frankenstein is forced to know the Creature he has spurned. Varieties of accusation, hatred, and remorse will pass between them. They will become one another's sole object of desire. But theirs is a meeting which is no meeting in the execution itself; they do not, cannot, know one another. In an excess of murder and vengeance, Frankenstein and his Monster will share only dread and despair. For the Creature's murderousness signifies the truth that life can never be restored to the dead, and the dead can never be restored to the living. Death is nature's absolute, and nature will brook no defiance. And so Frankenstein and his Creature die alone, unredeemed, and without hope of resurrection.

*Frankenstein* is an elucidation of love repudiated becoming hatred; of the humiliation that transmutes tenderness into vengeance. But this novel is more: it speaks of the malignant consequences of deny-ing death. For what, after all, is the crime that begets all others in *Frankenstein*? It is the insistence that death itself can be defeated: "Life and death appeared to me ideal bounds, which I should first break through, and pour a torrent of light into our dark world. A new species would bless me as its creator" (p. 53).

Frankenstein's signal crime is that he imagines himself to be larger than man and God and nature, that he refuses to accede to our "mortal coil." Like all those who take manic flight from death, Frankenstein has tasted loss and grief and desolation before he has fled them. His mother has recently succumbed to scarlet fever. Unconscious in his evasion of mourning, he becomes preoccupied with restoring life to the dead. Obsessed with his experiment, withdrawing from all human intercourse, the scientist "shunned my fellow creatures as if I had been guilty of some crime" (p. 55). Guilty, and yet ignorant of his true crime, he is the agent of his own tragic predicament. His refusal of death will only result in death's renewal. And his repudiation of his Creature will only make his Creature into a malignant icon of grief.

And so this chapter meditates on the crime that begets all oth-ers: Frankenstein's secession from life and his grandiose disputation of death. In the two years that have passed since his mother's death, Frankenstein's transactions have been exclusively with corpses: in charnel houses, in the plundering of graves. Constructing a creature from rank organs and body parts, Frankenstein experi-ences only awe for the product of his art. Intent on the restoration of life, he seems to adore the dead. For where is the horror that should attend such grim occupations? For Frankenstein, that horror does not attend the dismembering and theft of human limbs. Where an ordinary man might be roused to repulsion, Frankenstein is not. But he *is* roused to repulsion by the stirring of life within his creation. This, then, is the novel's central paradox, inviting curiosity and analysis: How is it that a Creature who was once beautiful as an inert composite of the dead, becomes hideous with the first breath of life? Frankenstein has sought to imbue his Creature with life; should not his success transport mere beauty into transcendence? But no:

His limbs were in proportion, and I had selected his features as beautiful . . . but these luxuriances only formed a
more horrid contrast with his watery eyes, that seemed
almost of the same colour as the dun white sockets in
which they were set, his shrivelled complexion and straight
black lips . . . the beauty of the dream vanished, and breath-
less horror and disgust filled my heart [p. 56].

What perversion finds the charnel house compelling, but is
horrified at the first emergence of life? What is the real nature of
the Creature's "ugliness"? I suggest that Frankenstein is repelled
because it is death *itself* that he has animated. Far from voiding
death, he has simply *given consciousness* to that which he had
denied. The Creature is an awakened corpse with eyes to see him,
a voice with which to command him, limbs with which to pursue him. And more: the Creature is the howling embodiment of
loss. For what a "birth" this is. At the very moment of his awakening, the Creature must look into the eyes of his maker's repug-
nance. And then, he is abandoned as the scientist flees from his
creation:

It was dark when I awoke; I felt cold also, and half frightened, . . . finding myself so desolate . . . I was a poor, helpless, miserable wretch; I knew, and could distinguish
nothing; but feeling pain invade me on all sides, I sat down
and wept [p. 103].

Filled with the desolation and grief that Frankenstein has disavowed in himself, the Creature exists in the borderland of the "it."
Neither human nor nonhuman, neither the living nor the dead,
bereft of all language and solace, he cannot escape from suffering.
Longing to be ushered into the human community, and forever
outside that communion, the Creature exists at the very apex of
loneliness. How strange that this "it" should go forth as the
embodiment of all human suffering, while Frankenstein, the man,
evades all the darkness in his soul. The Creature is the forgotten
relic of Frankenstein's grief. Because he can feel, the Creature

persists in seeking another whom he can love. When he cannot love and be loved, he will seek the other in destruction. Through vengeance upon Frankenstein, he will make his presence known.

> I gazed on my victim [Frankenstein's brother], and my heart swelled with exultation and hellish triumph: clapping my hands, I exclaimed, "I, too, can create desolation; my enemy is not invulnerable; *this death will carry despair to him*, and a thousand other miseries shall torment and destroy him" [pp. 143–144; italics added].

Where Frankenstein has forgotten his Creature, now he cannot but remember. Where he has disavowed loss, now loss will haunt him. The Creature entices him into a chase, inviting him to kill him if he is able. Frankenstein pursues him; he glimpses his Monster from afar, only to have his Monster elude him. The Monster is larger, faster, more powerful: Frankenstein has unleashed something he can no longer recapture, for "destiny was too potent, and her immutable laws had decreed my utter and terrible destruction" (p. 40). It is life and death that conform to immutable laws, it is loss that is too potent to be denied.

In the awareness of our own ending we find our humanity. Because he has risen from the dead and will return to the dead, because loneliness strikes him in the remembrance and anticipation of death, the Creature seems possessed of a human interior. As a purveyor of grief, he potentiates the restoration of Frankenstein's soul. But because he is a *malevolent* purveyor of grief, his own soul is forfeit. Tragic in its inception, *Frankenstein* is tragic in its ending, and the reader is left with the Monster's sorrow.

## FRANKENSTEIN'S FAMILIAL MEMORY AND THE COLLAPSE OF SUBJECTIVITY

How does Frankenstein become a man who cannot mourn? Shelley begins her novel in Frankenstein's childhood, which she casts as love's simple idyll. Shelley gives us the family Frankenstein:

kind, patient, and happily married parents; a playful younger brother named William; the tender, passively feminine Elizabeth, whom his parents adopted as a child and who becomes Frankenstein's betrothed-adoptive sister; and finally, their adored maid, Justine. Together they live an isolated country life, rich, fully sated in one another, absented from the world and from all human conflict. Characterized by fusion and stasis, it is a family of incestuous insularity. Everyone exists in a state of uncontested goodness. Individuation, interiority, conflict: these are occluded and diminished, ejected into the outside world. Goodness exists in the family's symbiosis; badness is imminent "out there." Although Frankenstein protests great love for all of his relations, his vision of them is attenuated: he sees them as his environment, as pleasing objects, as self-reflections. He does not know them as autonomously possessed of ambiguity and intention, conflict and interior. Empty of will, and without desire to be known, they seem pleased in their function as his environmental provision. Thus, he "looked upon Elizabeth as mine. . . . All praises bestowed on her, I received as made to a possession of my own" (p. 34), and Elizabeth seems content in this vision.

Life might be lovely, but then scarlet fever infects Elizabeth. In tending her daughter Elizabeth, who recovers, the mother dies. Even this mortal moment is cast as an idyll among idylls: "She died calmly and her countenance expressed affection even in death" (p. 42). Although she is terminally ill, we see neither her bodily pain nor her psychic suffering. It seems a death without dying. But her loss cannot be entirely evaded; familial bliss has been disrupted by the intrusion of death. Briefly they mourn, and this mourning precipitates the possibility of individuation: Frankenstein is encouraged to go away to school. He does not want to leave, but he accedes to his father's wishes.

He has felt his mother's loss: "I need not describe . . . the void that presents itself to the soul; and the despair that is exhibited on the countenance" (p. 42). But he desires forgetting, and cannot use grief to enrich his own interior. He yields to the mercies of Elizabeth, who tries to forget "even her own regret in her endeavors to make us forget" (pp. 42–43), for "memory brought madness with it" (p. 190). In this position, he departs for school, but he does not individuate. Unwilling to develop his own internal life, unwilling to recognize Elizabeth's autonomous evolution in his absence, his betrothal is an umbilical link to stagnation. Severed from his family, but denying the realities of loss and separation, he refuses the renewal of human interaction. He refuses to know his own loneliness: loneliness is the bad stuff of separation. He splits it off, and will projectively locate it inside his Creature, then sever all connection to that figure of loneliness. But loneliness will return as a persecutory object, thrusting upon Frankenstein all dimensions of human suffering.

One has the sense that Frankenstein cannot reengage the human world until he feels assured that relationships can occur without the other's leaving or *dying*. After his mother's death, he turns away from real human others and toward his experiment. He does not want to reengage with love until he knows that love will not be lost. He wants to reach inside of death and find a mother who cannot die. He wants a fungible mother endlessly replaced by mothers created by his own hands: she must cease her relentless dying. In trafficking with the dead, in mastering the life force, Frankenstein imagines that rotting limbs will cohere into immortality. It is this fantasized immortality that renders the inert Creature beautiful in his vision, so that "a resistless, and almost frantic, impulse urged me forward; I seemed to have lost all soul or sensation but for this one pursuit. . . . I collected bones from the charnel-houses and disturbed, with profane fingers, the tremendous secrets of the human frame" (p. 53).

But at last the Creature's eyes stir. In this stirring, Frankenstein understands that neither man nor God can excise separation from the human condition. In animating the dead, Frankenstein has not surpassed God in the creation of an infinite maternal mirror. He has rendered a Creature who has crossed over from the dead without forgetting the universe of death. This being is not a blank slate, void of memory and history, but a mordant Creature who has *his own agency and interior, a Creature that began in loss and is the living precipitant of loss*. It is loss and grief that cannot be borne, and from these Frankenstein takes flight. Once again he seeks to forget that pain which abides in the human condition: "'Why do you call to my remembrance,' I rejoined, 'circumstances of which I shudder to reflect'" (p. 100).

## FRANKENSTEIN'S CREATURE: SURVIVAL, REPARATION, AND THE FAILURE OF REPARATION

The moment of his birth is a moment of trauma, and so the Creature finds no solace in human recognition. Without resource or speech, the Creature seeks the warmth of another. But human encounter simply promises the renewal of annihilation. Cold, hungry, the Creature is ashamed of that ugliness which has alienated his maker. He wanders abroad by night, hiding his shame by day. At the same moment, Frankenstein lapses into fevered unconsciousness in a soft and feather bed. Frankenstein sleeps the sleep of oblivion, while his Creature cannot escape into forgetting. And when Frankenstein awakens, he is inauthentic with all who love him; he is secretive and tells no one of his experiment. Fraudulent with his family and suffocated by their shallow and ignorant love, their presence is nonetheless infected by Frankenstein's memory:

> I saw Elizabeth in the bloom of health. . . . Delighted and surprised I embraced her; but as I imprinted the first kiss on her lips they became livid with the hue of death; her features began to change, and I thought that I held the corpse of my death in my arms, a shroud enveloped her form [p. 47].

He tells them nothing, imagining that he can split his crime off from their goodness. His silence and avoidance potentiate evil's encroachment. When the Creature is still good, Frankenstein imagines him as evil. Frankenstein lives in persecutory anticipation, fearing the Creature's proximity. All malignance that lurks is attributed to his creation, while all goodness is retained within Frankenstein's family. Once obsessed with awakening the Creature, Frankenstein must now terminate the figure of that awakening:

first through disavowal, and later, by violence. The Creature is almost excised from human existence. Throughout most of the novel, the Creature is not clearly perceived. He is a shadow, obscured by storms and by darkness: "The figure passed me quickly, and I lost it in the gloom. . . . He soon reached the summit and disappeared. . . . The rain still continued and the scene was enveloped in an impenetrable darkness" (pp. 75–76).

Hurt and lost, visible only to himself, the Creature begins as the antithesis of malevolence. He searches for shelter, at last finding a hollow in the wall of a simple cottage. And through a hole in the wall, he has his first glimpse of human love, embedded in simple human memory. For therein lives a blind father, a son, a daughter. Poor, sad, hungry, and cold, they are tender with one another, ineffably linked in some mutually remembered tragedy. They have not cast mourning off from their memories; rather, mourning intensifies their bond. From his concealment, the Creature is moved, he has hope. Through watching this family, he learns speech, symbolization, and a sense of human history. And from them he learns the possibility of true bonding and human compassion. By night, the Creature cares for "his" cottagers: providing them with firewood, to warm them as they have warmed him. By day, he witnesses their mystified gratitude, and now feels the possibility of goodness within him. Here is his reparation for "offending" his maker. Here is his nascent depressive self. Now, the Creature conceives a plan: he will reveal himself to the blind man as the family's mysterious provider. Unable to perceive his hideous aspect, this kindly man might receive him into the human community, where the sighted only revile him. And so, the Creature waits until the blind father is alone, and enters the cottage. Just as the father begins to speak kindly to him, the rest of the family returns. Imagining the father is being attacked by the Creature, they scream. Abased, severed from depressive mutuality and from the recognition of his own goodness, the Creature flees those whom he has come to love.

So begins the Creature's experience of hate. All his efforts at love and reparation have failed; all expressions of tenderness are comprehended as violence, and so "evil became my good" (p. 219).

It is in the exhilaration of his murder of Frankenstein's young brother William that the Creature resolves to force his despair into Frankenstein's interior:

> Are you to be happy while I grovel in the intensity of my wretchedness? You can blast my other passions; but revenge remains, henceforth dearer than light or food! I may die, but first you, my tyrant and tormentor, shall curse the sun that gazes on your misery [p. 169].

## VENGEANCE AS BOND AND BONDAGE

Through this murder, Frankenstein is forced into a lived relation with the Creature he has forgotten; through it Frankenstein knows that "I had been the author of unalterable evil" (p. 92). And through this murder, the Creature emerges from obscurity to find himself face to face in a dialogue with his creator. Simultaneously wandering the countryside after the murder of William, Frankenstein and the Creature find one another. Speaking with the language he has acquired from his cottagers, the Creature reveals his soulfulness, his remorse, the degradation of human revilement. Immersed in his own rage and grief, no longer living at the surface of imaginary goodness, Frankenstein finally hears subjectivity speaking. For the first time, he is a human subject listening. And the Creature appeals to him:

> From you only could I hope for succor, although towards you I felt no sentiment but that of hatred. Unfeeling, heartless creator! You had endowed me with perceptions and passions, and then cast me abroad as an object for the scorn and horror of mankind. But on you only had I any claim for pity and redress, and from you I determined to seek that justice [p. 140].

The Creature asks Frankenstein to provide him with a female partner so that "I shall feel the affections of a sensitive being, and become linked to the chain of existence and events, from which I am now excluded" (p. 149). In the solace of a loving relation, he promises, all violence will cease. Temporarily resonant with the monster's plight and moved by the awareness of *his own responsibility*, Frankenstein agrees to create a partner for his Creature. Later, however, when they are apart, Frankenstein's paranoid–schizoid vision reasserts itself: he envisions monsters begetting monsters, ravaging those who are pure in their goodness. He then refuses to make a partner for his Creature, thereby stripping the beast of all reparative opportunity and insuring that its capacity for love will turn to vengeance. In the resurrection of the paranoid–schizoid modality, depressive subjectivity is once again eclipsed. Frankenstein can no longer see his Creature, and the Creature becomes invisible.

But the Creature refuses this invisibility. If he cannot be known and seen through love, then he must make himself visible through the sharing of loneliness. The Creature promises to annihilate everyone Frankenstein loves. As friends and relatives die, Frankenstein is no longer numb and no longer forgetting: "The blood flowed freely in my veins, but a weight of despair and remorse pressed on my heart, which nothing could remove. . . . Remorse extinguished every hope" (pp. 90–92). Thus the monster has pressed loneliness into Frankenstein's interior. The Creature assures that, one by one, Frankenstein's fraudulent relations fall away. When family and friends were alive, they refused to know Frankenstein's transgression. Now they are dead, and they have died without knowing. At last, Frankenstein and his Creature are alone with one another in a perverse but authentic discourse. Were the Creature not evil, there would be no connection. The Creature would have been forgotten, and the human condition would have been forgotten. Frankenstein would have resurrected his pale existence, chastely married to his "sister," never authentically encountering himself or another.

## DEATH, REMORSE, AND THE QUESTION OF REDEMPTION

But Frankenstein can never really know the autonomous experience of his benighted offspring. Instead of knowing him, he pursues him with murderous intent. And in a perverse quest for a reprieve from his loneliness, the Creature invites that murderous pursuit. And so this is their final attempt at dialogue: the Creature flees, Frankenstein pursues. And when Frankenstein falters, the Creature waits for him, coaxing him onward with signposts and portents. Eventually, Frankenstein is exhausted by the Creature's superhuman powers, much as he is morally exhausted by his own horror and hatred and remorse. Defeated, Frankenstein readies himself for death. At last he tells his story to a listener who empathizes *only with Frankenstein and not with the Monster*. Frankenstein dies, repentant and yet unrepentant: he never really recognizes his role in the Creature's malevolent transformation. When Frankenstein dies, the Creature realizes that Frankenstein is no longer pursuing him. Bereft, he seeks out his maker. Too late to witness Frankenstein's dying, the monster watches over the corpse. Always more possessed of a depressive self, it is the Creature who offers a soliloquy of repentance. Uttering "wild and incoherent self-reproaches," he recalls that

> a frightful selfishness hurried me on, while my heart was poisoned by remorse. Think you that the groans of Clerval [Frankenstein's best friend] were music to my ears? My heart was fashioned to be susceptible of love and sympathy; and when wretched by misery to vice and hatred it turned. It did not endure the violence of the change without torture such as you cannot even imagine . . . my pity amounted to horror; I abhorred myself [p. 218].

Penitent, robbed of his only intimate relation, and mournful for the murdered love within him, the Creature goes in search of his own death: "I shall no longer see the sun or stars, or feel the winds play on my cheeks. Light, feeling, and sense will pass away; and in this condition must I find my happiness" (p. 221). From corpses he was made and to a corpse he must return, filled with the remembrance and anticipation of death. And because he was imprisoned by Frankenstein's paranoid–schizoid vision, because he was never known as a human subject, the Creature's death will be inscribed on the sea, and never registered in human history:

> "I shall die . . . my ashes will be swept into the sea by the winds . . ." He sprang from the cabin-window, as he said this, upon the ice-raft which lay close to the vessel. He was soon borne away by the waves and lost in the darkness and distance [p. 221].

# CHAPTER 8

## THE PROBLEM OF REDEMPTION: FROM HOMICIDE TO PSYCHIC ANNIHILATION

IT WAS PRIOR TO THE ADVENT OF PSYCHOTROPIC MEDICATION. She was hospitalized after a suicide attempt. I was a new psychology extern. In the dayroom, patients masturbated and rocked; they muttered and screamed and grew violent. No one spoke anything recognizable as language. From this chaos I was to choose my first psychotherapy patients. Never had the therapeutic enterprise seemed so impotent and so absurd. Then I saw Pat. Massive, street-tough, and surly, she possessed a coherent wit and a sharp eye, as well as a strange sympathy for my naive intentions. Then, too, there was a certain mutuality of understanding: on this ward we were both disabled by futility. In our depression, we seemed matched across a great divide. And so, she spoke to me, seeking a reprieve from her loneliness, seeking a glimpse of another world, guiding me toward a modicum of therapeutic functioning. She was to be more effective with my depression than I was to be with hers.

Twice, then, I led her out of the dayroom, unlocked the ward's formidable steel door, and preceded her down a stairwell to a treatment room. This walk was silent. We passed no one. Twice, in our treatment room, she described her depression. Then, in our third session, she made her confession. Approximately six months prior to her hospitalization, she had committed a murder. Stoned on drugs, she had induced her White friends to murder a detested African-American hanger-on of their group. They overdosed their victim and waited for her to die. The victim struggled, and my patient strangled her. Marginal, poor, and unwanted, the victim and her death went unremarked by police.

She told it to me with a certain belligerent pride. She told it as sudden violence, with the brute force of intimidation. And she told it with the seductive intimacy of revelation. She told it as many things, but she did not tell it with remorse. And if she expressed no remorse for her act, so I expressed no explicit moral condemnation. I offered therapy as a curative space "free" from judgment. What then were we curing? For Pat, it was her depression; for me, it was her soul. But I was secret in my understanding. I imagined my task as the maintenance of analytic neutrality and "objectivity." But my own morality was implicit in transparent interpretations: I began to suggest that her depression and her attempted suicide were a manifestation of unexcavated guilt.

Through these interpretations (which may have captured an unconscious truth), I *imagined* her as remorseful, a suicidal penitent searching for punishment. In attributing morality to her prior to its existence, I filled her with human, depressive passions and eviscerated her bulk of its muscular volatility. I created an autistic monologue with her repentance, securely locating her murderous self in the past. In fact, she had no remorse. She claimed that the victim was a pestilence, now removed; drugs had merely disinhibited reasonable and expected street violence. To her, the depression bore no relation to the murder, but was the result of a broken relationship, and the loss of her foster child. Suicidal ideation was a manifestation of abandonment, not guilt. I refused to believe her. What did I know of the conditions of her street existence? I knew only my own just and sheltered universe. I *knew* she felt guilt: abandonment issues were secondary to this guilt; losses were experienced as retribution for her crime. I believed that she anticipated a life in which all attachments would rupture, as the "wheels of God grind slowly, and exceeding small."

And so, my presence in the therapeutic hour was fraught with contradiction. My interpretive set was an insistent condemnation of her act, as well as an insistent moral presumption. My demeanor of therapeutic neutrality and understanding was mendacious to its core; it belied the very content of my interpretations. I interpreted her guilt, yes, but I *behaved* as if I were present only as an agent of healing, as a purveyor of psychic absolution. I insisted on knowing her as a murderer no longer, but rather as a penitent who sought, and was entitled to, redemption and forgiveness.

I refused to know her as a murderess. I encountered her solely through the solipsism of my illusions, but my illusions did not conceal me from her perception. There was an aperture in our dissociative contagion, and through it she saw me, frightened, repulsed, filled with terrible human judgment. I could see her seeing me, and was shamed by the failure of my own therapeutic distance. Sometimes she pitied me, and sometimes she played me. She offered me her childhood, her nightmares and dreams. She entertained my suppositions. She would cry, and then seem to threaten me with violence. Back on the ward, she would protect me from other patients' physical and psychic assaults. I was grateful for her protection, and understood it as indicative of her native goodness. In truth, I was her possession; she could not allow me to figure in other patients' madness.

She was grateful for my companionship, but more, she was grateful for my terror. In that terror resided her only hope, for it was my only true knowledge of her condition. She was determined to foment this knowledge. In one session, she became angry and kicked me. Hard. Somehow my rage gained ascendancy over my terror. I leaped out of my chair and stood over her, yelling that she was a murderer, a menace, that she was never to touch me again. I shook my fist in her face. I was fed up with being bullied. (Perhaps another patient, a schizophrenic, had aided in my awakening: she had complained that Pat was just a "useless eater." Word salad, I thought, and then slowly thought again: of Pat, all hunger and envy and teeth, giving nothing, consuming everything, an amorphous bulk, fattening with cruelty while others grew lean with fear and deprivation. "Useless eater": not word salad, but succinct and penetrating, so unlike my convoluted, defensive analysis.) As I shook my fist, Pat stayed in her seat and took it. I felt a secret exultation. In her eyes I saw a moment of real contrition. I did not realize then the significance of her remaining seated. She wanted me to be bigger, outraged by her violence. She did not want the shallow, autistic presumption inherent in my civility and neutrality. She wanted to be *really real:* to be known and contained through my hatred (see Winnicott, 1949; Frederickson, 1990; Lionnells, 1997, personal communication). Only then could remorse begin to awaken. Briefly, our work became more collaborative and productive. The exploration of her childhood was more viscerally authentic.

But I was young, and I was in training. I understood that I had lost control of that pivotal session. To yell or to be physical toward a patient was anathema; to exult in such volatility, shameful. I must master the art of composure in extremity. If I had done things "right," she would not have kicked me. It was true that if I had done things "right," she might not have kicked me. I might not have shaken my fist in her face. But doing things "right" did not mean posing as neutral while concealing my morality in unempathic "objective" interpretations. I would not learn this lesson until much later.

I was young, and I neglected what she was trying to teach me. I repudiated confrontation and explicit moral condemnation, resumed my neutrality and the quest for "understanding," and retreated from our visceral exchange. In so doing, I resurrected my illusion, forcing on her my vision of her as a *murderer no longer.* In our brief confrontation I had finally allowed myself to know her as unrepentant, murderous in her potential. And yet, I had been strangely unafraid of being killed. In that moment, Pat's unrepentant murderer self shifted even as it was seen. She had felt hope and the possibility of redemption in a cycle of real human knowing and real human justice. Now, in the reconstitution of my analytic propriety, she found herself abandoned. In this transference–countertransference exchange, we lived the link between murder and loss. Ostensibly "forgiven" for her physical transgression against me, turned away from authentic reparative strivings toward the bland pursuit of "self-understanding," she was condemned to a lonely lifetime as a useless and murderous eater.

It was in this way that murder was linked to loss. Loss was an inevitability: it was not derived from guilt or from cosmic retribution. It was derived from a recurrent intersubjective failure. Her murderer self continually lost access to the other; it would not be known through the other's depressive hatred and concern. Insofar as another remained with her, her violence was denied. None but her criminal cohorts could meet her in her violence. And they were insensate to this violence; they could not meet her as she longed to be met. In the absence of an encounter with depressive hate and concern, she could not even locate that guilt which might then thirst for cosmic punishment. Thus, the resumption of my therapeutic politesse was not the resumption of proper therapeutic technique. It was a human failure, the preemption of the subject-to-subject dialogue of remorse and reparation. In the brevity of my rage, in the artifice of my forgiveness, I refused this murderer all possibility of redemption. When I left the hospital, she was still suicidal, and still an unrepentant killer.

## THE PROBLEM OF FORGIVENESS

> A few years back, a Tibetan monk who had served about 18 years in a Chinese prison in Tibet came to see me after his escape. . . . I had asked him what he felt was the biggest threat or danger while he was in prison. . . . He said that what he feared most was losing his compassion for the Chinese [Dalai Lama, 1998, pp. 129–130].

Granted: my forgiveness and my acceptance were a false edifice, constructed from fear, and loneliness, and appeasement, as well as from a student's reverential comprehension of the analytic situation. Perhaps my acceptance could have been made of finer stuff: not a pose, but a reservoir of strength and compassion; not a lie, but an embrace of the unrepentant as an accursed human other. If such forgiveness is possible, what is its promise? Does it precipitate atonement by the perpetrator and cleanse the victim's own interior? Does it transcend obscenity, as the Dalai Lama (1998) and Bishop Tutu (1998) suggest, or does it sanctify this obscenity? One wonders whether forgiveness will enable us to reclaim humanity, or merely incite evil with a permit for "cheap grace" (Tillich, as referenced by Pavlikowski, 1998). For if forgiveness offers cheap grace to the wicked, it can invite a "pitiless" abandonment of the victim (Ozick, 1998), a refusal to know that "the blood of the innocent cries forever" (S. Heschel, quoted in Ozick, 1998, p. 173).

For those who imagine forgiveness as transcendant (Dalai Lama, 1998; Tutu, 1998), compassion for one's enemy is absolute power against evil. From this perspective, goodness can never be vanquished because, as Martin Luther King said in 1963, "right temporarily defeated is stronger than evil triumphant" (p. 110). Here, one can suppose "that an act of forgiveness on our part could tip the scales toward compassion rather than brutality" (Brown, 1998, p. 123). But regardless of its effect on the perpetrator, some authors see the act of forgiveness as ennobling to the victim: it repudiates the hatred that reposes in the victim's interior (Enright, 1991); it liberates the victim from the bondage of vengeance (Pao, 1965); and it precipitates the reclamation of the victim's prior innocence. And if the victim can never return to an uncontaminated state, then at least the memory of horror can be transmuted into deeper wisdom. As one transmutes horror into wisdom, one repudiates the perpetrator's theft of one's soul.

One cannot dispute such healing possibilities. For some survivors, the very act of forgiving the unrepentant differentiates the good self from the bad perpetrator, thereby restoring a sense of benign human communion, and consolidating a sense of continuity with the pretraumatized self. In the labyrinth of good and evil, there are no singular prescriptions for either perpetrator or victim. As Safer (1999) and Tutu (1998) suggest, the act of forgiveness can heal or it can violate. But wherever forgiveness transpires without a dialogue with the perpetrator's repentance, it remains linked to trauma's solitude:

Deciding whether to forgive is one of the loneliest tasks in the world. It is most often performed in solitude surrounded only by memories, in dialogue with yourself and those who are gone, torn between the longing to understand and overcome the pain and the dread of obliterating its meaning, wondering whether to annihilate love or to resurrect it [Safer, 1999, p. 7].

If we understand the nucleus of evil as catastrophic loneliness, the forgiveness of evil will inevitably be lonely. And yet, ideally, authentic forgiveness should be an organic *intersubjective* process. It should be a lived dialogue between perpetrator, bystander, and victim; it should be a dialogue that both alleviates and confirms catastrophic loneliness. Authentic forgiveness cannot be coerced by family, culture, or analyst. Where it is an organic process, forgiveness is not linked to forgetting. But where the culture presses the victim to forgive, it usually exhorts him to *forget:*

> And I,
> I forget to be Negro in order to forgive
> No longer will I see my blood upon their hands
> it's sworn. . . .
>
> I forget to be Negro to forgive the world for this
> [U'Tamsi on the murder of Emmett Till, quoted in Soyinka, 1999, p. 120].

And forgetting is the first condition of evil's dissociative contagion. To many victims of heinous crimes, forgiveness does not restore their interior but violates it. Although theologians such as the Dalai Lama and Bishop Tutu pointedly differentiate forgiveness and forgetting, for many survivors, forgiveness *is* an abandonment of memory. As such, it is an invitation to dissociation and to the renewal of destruction. For these survivors (and for those who have not survived), "The face of forgiveness is mild, but how stony to the slaughtered" (Ozick, 1998, p. 217). As Soyinka (1999) suggests, it is not forgiveness but "justice [that] constitutes the first condition of humanity . . . justice assigns responsibility" (p. 31) and requires some reparation and restitution. In the most malevolent cases, rather than being forgiven, humanity will tend to hold the perpetrator outside of the human circle. There, the perpetrator is relentlessly alone, never absolved of "the indissoluble bond fusing the criminal to the crime" (Langer, 1998, p. 187). He is met only in humanity's curse:

> Let the SS man die unshriven
> Let him go to hell.
> Sooner the fly to God than he
> [Ozick, 1998, p. 220].

And this curse may obtain for the penitent as well as the unrepentant:

> We condemn the brute; he is a barbarian; we condemn him as we condemn every barbarian. How then can we dare to condemn the man of conscience, as if there was no difference between him and the barbarian.

> We condemn the intelligent man of conscience because there *is* a difference, because though at heart not a savage, he allowed himself to become one, he did not resist. It was not that he lacked conscience; he smothered it. It was not that he lacked sensitivity; he coarsened it. It was not that he lacked humanity, he deadened it [Ozick, 1998, p. 219].

This rage is that "medicine" which Macduff calls upon as the "cure for this deadly grief" (*Macbeth*, act 4, scene 3). It is what Liegner (1980) describes as "the hate that cures." But this same hate, seemingly so antithetical to compassion and redemption, frequently offers the perpetrator an authentic human engagement, critical to his containment and to his own process of redemption. It may be the only form of authentic communication such a patient can hear (Bach, 1994). From the time of the Psalms to Shakespeare to present psychoanalytic theory, there is some understanding that hate may evoke a moral awakening in the perpetrator:

> I know what Transgression says to the wicked;
> he has no sense of the dread of God,
> because its speech is seductive to him
> till his iniquity be found out and he be hated
> [Psalm 36, verse 2]

and that reparation and restitution are prerequisites to the perpetrator's redemption:

> O, my offense is rank, it smells to heaven.
> . . . . . . . . .
> A brother's murder. Pray can I not,
> Though inclination be as sharp as will.
> My stronger guilt defeats my strong intent,
> . . . . . . . . .
> My fault is past. But, O, what form of prayer
> Can serve my turn? "Forgive my foul murder"?
> That cannot be, since I am still possessed
> Of those effects for which I did the murder,
> My crown, mine own ambition, and my queen.
> May one be pardoned and retain th' offense?
> [*Hamlet,* act 3, scene 3].

## OBJECTIVE HATRED VERSUS THE PROBLEM OF VENGEANCE

To condemn and not to forgive. To condemn and later, to forgive. To hate, and to get over hating. Such positions provide the perpetrator with an encounter with "objective hatred" (Winnicott, 1947); they call on him to make reparation to the other whom he has violated. And through objective hatred, he comes to know that his destructiveness is contained, that it will no longer annihilate the innocent. And this "objective hatred" which seeks justice and contains evil, may even potentiate remorse. These themes are most fully articulated by Winnicott:

> [I]n certain stages of certain analyses the analyst's hate is actually sought by the patient, and what is then needed is hate that is objective. If the patient seeks objective or justified hate he must be able to reach it, else he cannot feel that he can reach objective love [1947, p. 199].

These themes are also expounded by Coltart (1986) and Frederickson (1990). Coltart (1986), Pao (1965), and Rappaport (1998) describe clinical moments when they angrily resign from the patient's destructive usage of them. In such moments, "the analyst has shown himself to be capable of standing apart from and opposed to some of the lethally persecutory and oppressive aspects of the patient's personality" (Rappaport, 1998, p. 375), and this stance often precipitates change. While Slochower (1996) and Epstein (1977, 1984) do not advocate confronting the patient with the analyst's objective hatred, neither do they suggest retaining interpretation's air of benign neutrality. Slochower suggests a form of "holding" in which the patient hears her own impact in the analyst's tough voice and in her limit-setting demeanor. Whether the analyst utilizes Slochower's form of holding, or more confrontational interpersonal techniques, the analyst informs the destructive patient that annihilation is refused, that destructiveness will be contained, that the analyst will survive and will insure that others will survive.

From this perspective, I am opposed to the forgiveness of the unrepentant; I believe it facilitates malignant dissociative contagion and evil's reproduction. I am opposed to any form of analytic moral neutrality that appears to offer moral acceptance or absolution for the patient's malevolence. The therapist needs to recall that, in Schafer's (1983) words: "It is not a departure from neutrality to call a spade a spade" (p. 4). Indeed, as Greenberg (1999) redefines analytic neutrality, it "embodies the goal of establishing an optimal tension between the tendency to see the analyst as an old object and his capacity to experience him as a new one" (p. 142).

In general, the analyst encountering evil must act as a new object, one who demonstrably occupies a different moral universe than the patient's old objects. If, as Greenberg notes, silence and anonymity tend to allow the analyst to be experienced as an old object, and activity establishes the analyst as a new one, then I must argue for activity in the presence of malignance.

To convey object-related hatred for the malevolent act is to function as a new moral object. This functioning potentiates the patient's shift toward true mutuality and empathic resonance with the other. Whether we are working with the survivor or we are working with the perpetrator (or bystander), the implied neutral acceptance of the unrepentant is a solipsistic process, problematic in its sheer autism. It is not an intersubjective dialogue in which the perpetrator's guilt and the victim's annihilation are mutually recognized. Forgiveness/acceptance of the unrepentant is a monologue, in which the monologue of forgiveness mirrors the perpetrator's monologue of torture: it is another collapse of intersubjectivity. Where the perpetrator was previously encapsulated in his fantastic malignant enactment, now he is encapsulated in the fantastic reprieve of love and absolution. Culpability remains occluded and he is never required to meet the real other, or to know himself as real. To embrace the unrepentant perpetrator in the soft envelope of forgiveness is to abandon the perpetrator to the loneliness of his own depravity. And, in its failure of intersubjective recognition, such forgiveness/acceptance also represents a failure of historical inscription: the perpetrator is never seen in execution's moment—not in the moment when he himself was annihilated, nor in the moment when he annihilates another. While some perpetrators may be touched by their victim's immeasurable goodness, locating remorse *because* they have already been forgiven, the monologue of forgiveness/acceptance rarely invites such transformation. Generally, undeserved forgiveness escalates the perpetrator's destructive striving to be known and seen in the execution itself. Fenichel (1928) notes this impossible predicament, as he quotes a patient who alternates between sadism and masochism: "I will murder them all, and then at least I shall be put in prison, and shall not need a neurosis any longer" (p. 53).

When the perpetrator is not seen through condemnation, nothing contains him. When he is not contained, he cannot be redeemed. Condemnation, justice, reparation: these are the first conditions for the perpetrator's restraint and redemption. The leit-motif of this book, then, is: for the perpetrator to be known and redeemed, his crimes must be met by a psychoanalytic culture of object-related hatred. Such a culture (derived from the "depressive mode" discussed in chapter 5) insists on the perpetrator's knowl-edge of his crimes. It does not promise absolution, rather it strives toward the intersubjective recognition (see Benjamin, 1988) of the guilty and the innocent. It does not promise redemption, but offers opportunities for reparation. Object-related hatred retains a vision of the perpetrator as a whole object: it regards the most heinous crime as the inhuman act of a human soul. This mode of address allows the culture to hate and to get over hating (see Galdston, 1987); it allows us to imagine revenge and to abandon revenge (Akhtar, 1999) in favor of justice. And insofar as this type of hate links the past and the future (Pao, 1965), it facilitates evil's historical inscription, thereby defying evil's erasure of its history.

But, as Van Zyl (1999) and Straker suggest in their eloquent neo-Kleinian discussion of the Truth and Reconciliation Committee in South Africa, the pursuit of justice must be distinguished from the pursuit of vengeance. In the aftermath of atrocity, murder, life-long racism, or familial abuse, the victim's thirst for vengeance may never subside. Nonetheless, we must restrain that vengeance which merely reproduces the evil it seeks to avenge. Vengeance, unlike object-related hatred, is a sadistic manic defense (see chapters 5 and 6); it flees mourning and hopelessness, and denies trauma's irre-trievable loss (Horney, 1948; Searles, 1956; Socarides, 1966; Van Zyl, 1999). It is grounded in oblivion and denial, and stands opposed to the awakened knowledge of evil's history. As such, vengeance is an agent of malignant dissociative contagion, not its adversary. The avenger maintains the very bondage that oppresses him (Socarides, 1966); he cannot separate from his perpetrator, nor align himself with the just. The punishments he conceives are sadistic in intent; they induce shame rather than guilt (see Gilligan, 1992). Insofar as they abase, they consolidate the cycle of evil, resulting in the renewal of crime (Fenichel, 1925; Gilligan, 1992). In pursuit of such punishments, the avenger assumes a pseudo-courageous aspect: revenge is sought against all odds, regardless of risk (Pao, 1965). This false moral courage is a mere simulation of justice, in which the avenger "attempts to masquerade as his victim's superego" (Socarides, 1966, p. 371), rather than evoking the awakening of the perpetrator's own superego. In contrast, object-related hatred requires authentic courage; it punishes but does not humiliate. It provides opportunities for the perpetrator to make reparation; it affirms the perpetrator who has found remorse, and who is willing to make restitution to the human community. Condemnation, justice, reparation, redemption: these potentiate a subject-to-subject dialogue. Vengeance, humiliation, violation, cruelty: these reproduce evil.

## REDEMPTION AND THE PERSISTENCE OF MEMORY

In a just culture, in which the perpetrator is contained as a *depraved human subject*, the perpetrator may come to long for redemption. To find redemption, a perpetrator must despair of absolution. Relinquishing all claims to forgiveness, faithful to guilt and to memory, he must turn away from himself toward the other, committing himself to a life of restitution and reparation. In his remorse, through long acts of reparation, he may find redemption and even absolution. If he finds this reprieve, he finds it through the slow embrace of the human community, an embrace characterized at least as much by rage as it is by forgiveness. It is repentance that precedes all possibility of redemption, and it is reparation that transforms guilt into wisdom. Forgiveness is not the perpetrator's entitlement. When it occurs, it is a gift of extraordinary humanity: it is a recognition of transformation, of the authenticity of remorse, of the desire to make reparation. And where it cannot occur, this too is a perverse gift of human communion: here the perpetrator's crime is met and known as irredeemable.

Even if condemnation and justice inspire repentance, and even if repentance inspires forgiveness, the perpetrator may never again feel that he is cast in love's simple light. He is never freed from the confinement of memory:

> My moral guilt is not subject to the statute of limitations, it cannot be erased in my lifetime [but] . . . I looked into your eyes, eyes that reflected all the murdered people, eyes that have witnessed the misery, degradation, fatalism and agony of your fellow human beings . . . when we parted, you wrote for me in my copy of your book that I did not repress that ruthless time, but had recognized it responsibly in its true dimensions. . . . Every human being has his burden to bear. Noone can remove it for another, but for me, ever since that day, it has become much lighter [Speer, 1998, pp. 245–246].

In his victim's eyes, the repentant perpetrator may find exquisite moments of mutuality. But even as the perpetrator finds such moments, he must inevitably succumb to the loneliness of memory. This memory perpetually casts aspects of his perpetrator self outside of the human circle, even as he is received back into it. The perpetrator can never fully reenter the human circle, because the perpetrator self who committed the transgression is never the self who repents and is forgiven. This perpetrator self exists somewhere beyond intersubjective recognition; it can be signified only through the rupture of mutuality. Like the survivor, the perpetrator will always possess an area of self experience that is beyond mutual knowing. The human comfort of forgiveness may be proffered and received, but no one can fully absolve the perpetrator's guilt nor eradicate his history.

Whether a crime is heinous or the transgression is mild, there is something inevitably tragic in this dynamism of redemption. Never purely transcendant, but always scarred with despair, redemption recapitulates annihilation's paradox: it begins alone, becomes a search for mutuality, and then collapses backwards into solitude. Here, as in trauma survival, the private core of pain and death is registered through the rupture of human relatedness, through the impenetrability of human isolation. This dynamism exists even when the crime is not monstrous, but ordinary, human, eminently forgivable. It exists wherever the transgressor's history of annihilation is reproduced through another's pain. And so, I end with a case of mild transgression, of the sort that daily enters our office. Not murder, not "evil," but a narcissistic exploitation and extinction of another's self: it was a "crime" so mild and unintended, a trespass so readily forgiven, that its tragic dimension seemed like a perverse revelation of the human condition.

## FALSE GUILT, FALSE FORGIVENESS, AND THE TRAGEDY OF REAL REDEMPTION

It was a treatment that began with one kind of death and ended in another. They came in, carrying the stillbirth of their sexuality silently between them. Not yet old enough to consign sexuality to the ashes, they came, but they came without hope. They were earthy, dynamic, and vitally engaged with living. She was an artist and an activist working on behalf of abused women. He was the rock of his community: an ordinary man dispensing extraordinary kindness. And yet, the deep interior of their marital relation was vacant, emptied of life. It was as if they were left alive in a nuclear desert, wandering listlessly and alone after the conflagration. She was an incest survivor. They had not had sex in many years. Theirs was a kindly marriage, cooperative, responsible; it was devoid of sexual gesture, of lived color, of controversy, of all intimate connection. Inert and still, they lived entirely without hatred or desire. Their sexuality reminded me of the words of A. Brink (1982), speaking of a township laid waste by apartheid:

> For twenty years this whole area had been lying fallow, scarred and exposed; . . . and still the disfiguring wound lay visible, uncured, incurable, like earth on which the devil had left his imprint, causing everything to wither and die, forever barren. . . . What had prompted them to come here, today of all days? There was nothing here. Only the wind [p. 46].

To be with this couple inside their marital relation was to be drawn into a wasteland in which one's very mind and limbs seemed paralyzed and each moment's lived experience evaporated into oblivion.

The psychoanalytic discovery of her incest story had been evocative of great pain and revelation and had healed many somatic complaints—her depersonalization, her fractured self-esteem, and her states of panic—and it had enhanced her engagement with living. But a myriad of therapies had ultimately met the blunt intractability of her sexual shame and terror; it would not yield. Sexually, she metabolized nothing, desired nothing. Mind closed, vagina closed, her sexuality eluded penetration and found death. Having long ago repudiated the female self who experienced annihilating incestuous eroticism, her body became a ruined and melancholy landscape. With arousal signifying culpability and disintegration, all agency was disavowed (Ehrenberg, 1987; Lionells, 1997). She could not locate herself as an agent of resistance or as an agent of desire. Her body was a living, inviolable protest against child rape, and yet the protest implicit in her body's resistance was perpetually dissociated. It was not really real and not really *hers*; *she* was not angry; *she* wanted to have sex for her husband's sake but *could not*. The secret terrorism of her resistance was a shape shifter, fluid and invisible, finding personification in myself, her analyst, her husband, her marital operations, and her own psychosomatic complaints. She transformed her therapies into a series of abortive rapes in which she was neither responsible for sexuality nor for its refusal: we were to force her to become sexual, and then find ourselves castrated by the *dissociated strength of her own resistance*. We were the perpetrator, and we lived the perpetrator's imperative defeat. But in our defeat she could find no victory or exaltation. Her life was one of protest, but in the arena of her own body, she steadfastly relinquished her own defiance. As therapy after therapy failed to awaken her sexuality, she remained shamed, guilty, remorseful. Neither woman nor child, victim or agent, she was a wretched *thing*, familiar only with failure and abasement.

To speak with this couple of sexuality was to enter an impossibility; all such dialogue collapsed into the bottomless well of the wife's traumatic affect. The therapeutic field was entirely consumed by the wife's guilt, shame, and terror; her tears eclipsed her husband's voice. She was angry at no one, critiqued no one. Beneath the wrenching affective resonance of her incest memory there existed within and between husband and wife an interminable silence and stagnation, embedded within a subtle relation of dominance and submission. He was intelligent, quiet; empathically receptive toward her grief but ineffectually engaged in their joint struggle toward sexuality. He listened but did not enquire; he gently comforted but did not act; he supported, but would neither protect nor intervene. He had met the long years of their sexual paralysis with passive resignation, ostensibly deferring to her pain, leaving her to initiate and sustain all therapeutic intervention. He was not angry in or for himself. He knew that *she* needed to locate *her* lost rage at her parental tormentors. Every few years he voiced a quiet frustration, a muted rage at her parents for the damage they inflicted upon *her*. His own interior was a cipher, absent and invisible. Remarkably complacent in his invisibility, he continually vanished in his mute capitulation to her trauma. In session, he eluded even the gentlest probe of his own feelings, and particularly, of his own family history, claiming it was forgotten, irrelevant. For him, being psychodynamically known seemed to signify the annihilating rupture of a fragile self. In the prevailing flood of her traumatic affects, he located both the despair of sexual fulfillment, and the welcome shelter of his own obscurity. Saintly and eviscerated, he enveloped her frigidity in a shallow forgiveness. He knew and forgave the *wrong* "crime": the absence of sex deflected him from her plundering of his soul. She stole his self, and he abdicated his self. And he subsisted in the dream of grafting hot desire onto empty self-abnegation.

She was lost in his forgiveness. It offered her no contours, no containment or resistance. The abyss of her remorse expanded but never found authenticity: she gnawed grievously on her sexual incapacity and never knew herself as the agent of his annihilation. The more she gnawed, the more he forgave. The more he forgave, the more her guilt reached suicidal proportions. He would not know the killing field of their relation, and so she signaled it with her imagery of death. She longed for his knowing, his rage, and his refusal of her trespass. Only then could she be known. Only then would the perpetrator find constraint, releasing her to exult in the potency of her sexual repudiation of her husband.

But she could not sustain the relational space in which he could reach that liberating objective hatred. She was fearful of his nascent self and its potentially annihilating eclipse of *her* soul. She loved him. But she was vigilant in her repression of his interior. She continually disrupted my efforts to find his inner life by flooding the field with traumatic affect in those rare moments of his subjective, autonomous emergence. Before the cataclysmic force of incest, his tenuous feelings and gestures fell away. With his invisibility resurrected, she insured his disappearance, even as she sustained his fragile self through its concealment. In their joint reconstitution of his obscurity and passivity, she would then find herself abandoned, bereft of his strength and protection, alone with trauma's stigmata. She was once again a child without rescue, a perpetrator without restraint. She would dream of her husband's passivity in the face of imminent danger. In these dreams, she was both perpetrator and victim, alone in all attempts to rescue her own children.

She was not angry at his passivity. He was not angry at being silenced. She engaged in a recurrent traumatic abreaction that changed nothing. He engaged in an empathic forgiveness that cured nothing. Her history of incest gave her exclusive rights to an internal life. His forgiveness gave him exclusive rights to goodness. In many ways she was a nurturer and an advocate, both to him and to the needy and the abused, but she could not know herself in her own goodness. She knew herself only as a bad wife who withheld something essential from a man impeccable in his goodness. He was confident of his goodness, but did not know *who* it was that was good. He did not imagine that he tormented her with the falsity of his forgiveness, that he abandoned her with his vacuity. He missed sex but did not miss the self who would have sex. He was a man without history or context, without a desire to be found or known. He knew himself, and was known by her, as an object to her as subject. She was his speech, his shape, his form, his meaning; he was her silence, her absence, her sacrifice, her eternal submission. She could not be located in the transference play of his childhood, only he could be located in hers. He is her child-self, mute, an orifice to be filled with parental madness. He is also the castratus, the father-perpetrator, now prone and submissive, upon whom *she* performs rape. But she cannot hear the answering agony of his rage and terror. There is no meeting. They have one self between them, and it is hers.

This dynamism possesses the stasis of death. In it, he and she are devoid of all struggle and have collapsed the dynamic separation that gives rise to nonincestuous sexuality. I am concerned less with the absence of sex than with the absence of his self. I begin to limit the time devoted to her repetitive incestuous abreaction. I inquire into his life's concerns like a nonincestuous parent interested in the ordinariness of childhood. We speak of sports, of finances, of office politics. She interrupts, deflects: this is an evident waste of time. I insist, and she suffers it, bewildered, inattentive, like a narcissistic mother lost in her own preoccupations. She restrains herself, like an incestuous father in the daytime, ever confident of night's promised obscurity and its license of perversion. Through the ordinariness of his life he begins to reveal himself: his strength and fear of assertion and conflict, his confusion over his feelings, his tendency to relinquish his own needs, particularly his anger. I can sense her raging in her confinement.

Then her body begins speaking through the resurgence of long absent somatic complaints: headaches, vaginal pain, weakness in her legs. She is depressed, anxious. He is attentive and kind, and he goes into retreat, hiding himself to take care of her. I support his kindness and concern, but I do not allow him his invisibility. I insist he continue speaking. He complains that she is never strong enough to support him in his life's anxieties, that she always requires his care. This time, he says, he wants her to be strong enough for him in a serious career crisis he is undergoing. He does not want to have to defer his needs to take care of her again. I realize that I am hearing his anger, individuation, and desire: he now resists her annihilation of his interior. This is his first voice of object-related hatred.

I suggest ways she can care for herself, and be cared for, tolerating her own states while nonetheless considering his needs. She, who is always "nice," yells, *"You can't make me, no one can make me, I'm sick of being forced, I won't do it,"* and leaves the session. Nonplussed but impressed, he knows this is the lost voice of her childhood protest, which he has long awaited. This rage has never been manifest in her perseverative incest narrative. Nonetheless, he is still angry on his own behalf. They are now two selves in conflict. This explosive therapeutic interaction is repeated several times: each time, she finds that she is not abandoned, but rather is encouraged in her expression of dormant incestuous rage. At the same time, he is encouraged to persist in pursuing his own needs and feelings, and she is required to consider them. Through her body symptoms I have heard her dissociated resistance, and then, he states her split off childhood protest to her perpetrator: *I don't care how damaged you are, you must consider me, care for me, and not disregard me.* She experiences his assertion as a requirement to submit to the man's perverse needs. They cannot both exist. Someone must be extinguished. Perhaps my office can provide a new space, in which no one will be permitted to annihilate and no one will submit to annihilation.

In therapy, no one annihilates and no one submits. Their relation is newly imbued with mutual conflict. In his anger, he is no longer the sole possessor of goodness; she is no longer the sole possessor of self. When she abuses, she is not lost in his vacuity: she is found in his "objective hatred." When she rages, he does not abandon her, but instead he is enlivened and demanding. There follows a period of playful sexual flirtation. I am with a man and a woman teasing one another. He gives her flowers, jewelry. She gives him the gift of a sexual dream she has had about him. He is charmed. They watch romantic movies, take long walks, leave the children at home. They remember the early days of their love, a snowstorm, making love before a fire. They laugh. They do not touch sexually, but we can all feel that imminent possibility. And as they play at this possibility, so his being comes more sharply into focus. Suddenly, he has a history, stories from the past: old girlfriends, odd sexual predicaments suggestive of his own inhibitions.

The stories are factual, laced with amusement and some disappointment. There is still no reflection, little sense of an internal life; he is without emotional memory or childhood context. But he does offer us sketches of home: his mother, his father, his brother. He cannot stop speaking, and she is absorbed, attentive. He senses that his stories have meaning, and hopes to have that meaning discovered in our listening. He is quietly charming, and looking rather more handsome.

They are becoming disembedded, two selves, sometimes meeting in opposition, sometimes in differentiated, loving mutuality. Although he has just barely emerged, she is no longer annihilating his interior. He is stronger with her and for her, more proactive. Each of them is becoming more empowered in their goodness, relinquishing their saintly and demonic pretensions. Where they formerly existed in islands of neglect, now they evolve a truer friendship. She evolves a compassionate consideration of his needs in relation to herself, experiencing remorse for having consumed him. Having been angry, and having received her authentic remorse, he can now forgive her for her real "crime." Having becoming loving, she can now require him to examine his collusion in his own evisceration. At times, she still seeks to consume him, and still he retreats into invisibility. But now, she sometimes meets his anger and persistence; his anger releases her own rage at her own perpetrator. The therapeutic atmosphere is one of warmth and humor and mutual assistance; I feel awake and facilitating where I had felt nullified and dead. I even imagine their sexual restoration.

At this juncture, death's shadow fell upon their liberation: at the very moment of their imminent sensuality, his body became ill. The somatic symptoms that had fallen silent in her body seemed to relocate themselves in his. Previously athletic and robust, his teeth, joints, and heart began to fail. Innocuous at first, his symptoms became increasingly ominous. Playful sexuality was displaced by grief and terror; individuation was lost to a sense of his bestial degradation. It was as if the persistence of traumatic memory took up residence in his viscera, extinguishing *his* emergent "heart." Heart disease and medical interventions assumed the implacable aspect of her incestuous experience: invasive, agonizing, degrading events in which he was forced to submit in order to survive. These same medical interventions assumed the hope and the impotence of a child's resistance.

The course of his illness was one year. In that year, he succumbed to death and found the ultimate voice of his own resistance. He discovered his autonomous psychic life, long dormant affects and vulnerabilities, his own childhood history of which he had never spoken. He spoke of his own feelings and needs, expressed his longings, his desire for comfort. He remembered his father's embrace, and the early rupture of that embrace. He longed for his father's arms around him, and asked his children for physical tenderness. They gave it, and he felt his father return. He awakened in his family a deep sense of intimacy, and led them in confronting their grief. His community acknowledged him for his lifelong kindness, generosity, and wisdom: he wept, knowing himself in his real *earthly* goodness. He felt deeply that his life had been meaningful.

In the frailty of his body, in the emergence of his fear and sorrow, she was tender, resourceful, kind. His death was the measure of her solitude. Her acts of reparation both comforted and failed him. She feared that her nascent sexuality had murdered him. She sensed that she offered him solace in his pain. She believed that her own resurrection must always be confounded with death. But now, in the care of his dying, her survivor self made reparation for the bestial gestures of her survival; her perpetrator self made reparation to her beloved husband. She came to know him *in and for himself*. She was his father's arms around him, embracing her beloved as he died. He was full with his inner self as he lay dying. Their most exquisite intimacy was located, not in sexuality, but in the long moments of his body's disintegration.

In that last year, I finally knew him. He revealed himself to me, and taught me to comfort him. I miss him. I wonder if I will die as well. I miss her. I wonder if I will comfort my husband as well in his final illness. I said goodbye to my patient in his coffin. He did not look like himself. There was the mournful exaltation of his crowded wake, and there were the lonely limits of that exaltation. No one could die his death for him. No one could grieve his wife's solitary grief. No one returned with me to an office made still and silent by death. I have thought many times of the two of them: her violation and his surrender, his refusal and her redemption; the perverse autonomy of death as it defined her resurrection.

## CONCLUSION

Protest-condemnation-repentance-reparation-forgiveness-redemption: this is a cycle that celebrates mankind's capacity for goodness. It is a cycle that contains and repudiates moral transgression, but cannot entirely arrest evil's reproduction. As long as trauma is a death died alone, as long as pain has no words to convey itself to another, evil will register the contradictory desires of catastrophic loneliness. Despite the power of art and the testimonials of justice, despite the tenderness of reparation and the mutuality of redemption, the primal fragmentation of extinction finds historical registration only in a *violating rupture of human contact.* A new victim will be reduced to an "it."

But if the allegiance to memory and to history inspires evil, so it inspires good. Neither good nor evil exists in autonomous pure forms, as the victorious in relation to the vanquished. Rather, good and evil define one another. Awesome in their powers, deriving meaning in their struggle for ascendancy, and urgency from their contest with death, good and evil will always meet one another to define the human condition.

As psychoanalysts encountering both good and evil, we must "hold" (see Slochower, 1996) both hope and despair. We must act on behalf of good and against evil. We must praise justice, and seek justice, because "with this faith we will be able to hew out of the mountain of despair a stone of hope" (King, 1963, p. 105). We commit to hope, knowing it will give way to despair; we commit to historical subjectivity, knowing it will yield to amnesia. Here, in this tension, traumatic memory exists, reasoned and irrational, civilized and yet left alone in the wilderness beyond knowing. Here, traumatic memory cries out to the last:

If thou didst ever hold me in thy heart,
Absent thee from felicity awhile,
And in this harsh world draw thy breath in pain,
To tell my story.

. . . . . . . .

the rest is silence
[*Hamlet,* act 5, scene 2].

# REFERENCES

Abel, G. G., Gore, D., Holland, C., Camp, N., Becker, J. & Rathner, J. (1989), The measurement of the cognitive distortions of child molesters. *Annals Sex. Res.*, 2:135–153.

Akhtar, S. (1999), Hatred. In: *Inner Torment*. Northvale, NJ: Aronson.

Alford, C. F. (1997), *What Evil Means to Us*. Ithaca, NY: Cornell University Press.

Alford, C. F. (1998), Melanie Klein and the nature of good and evil. In: *Psychoanalytic Visions of the Human Condition: Philosophies of Life and Their Impact on Practice*, ed. P. Marcus & A. Rosenberg. New York: New York University Press, pp. 118–140.

Alpert, J. L. (1994), Analytic reconstruction in the treatment of an incest survivor. *Psychoanal. Rev.*, 2:217–235.

Alpert, J. L. (1997), Story-truth and happening-truth. In: *Memories of Sexual Betrayal*, ed. R. Gartner. Northvale, NJ: Aronson, 1997.

Amery, J. (1995), Torture. In: *Art from the Ashes*, ed. L. Langer. Oxford: Oxford University Press, pp. 121–138.

Arendt, H. (1955), *Men in Dark Times*. New York: Harcourt Brace Jovanovich.

Arendt, H. (1963), *Eichmann in Jerusalem: A Report on the Banality of Evil*. New York: Penguin Books.

Aron, L. (1996), *Mutuality in Psychoanalysis*. Hillsdale, NJ: The Analytic Press.

Auerhahn, N. C. & Laub, D. (1987), Play and playfulness in holocaust survivors. *The Psychoanalytic Study of the Child*, 42:45–58. New Haven, CT: Yale University Press.

Bach, S. (1994), *The Language of Perversion and the Language of Love*. Northvale, NJ: Aronson.

Balint, M. (1968), *The Basic Fault*. New York: Brunner/Mazel.

Barton, C. A. (1993), *The Sorrows of the Ancient Romans: The Gladiator and the Monster*. Princeton, NJ: Princeton University Press.

Baumeister, R. F. (1997), *Evil: Inside Human Violence and Cruelty*. New York: W. W. Freeman.

Becker, E. (1973), *The Denial of Death*. New York: Free Press.

Becker, E. (1975), *Escape from Evil*. New York: Free Press.

Beebe, B. & Lachmann, F. M. (1988), Mother–infant mutual influence and precursors of psychic structure. In: *Frontiers in Self Psychology: Progress in Self Psychology, Vol. 3*, ed. A. Goldberg. Hillsdale, NJ: The Analytic Press, pp. 3–25.

Benjamin, J. (1988), *The Bonds of Love*. New York: Pantheon Books.

Benjamin, J. (1995), *Like Subjects, Love Objects: Essays on Recognition and Sexual Difference*. New Haven, CT: Yale University Press.

Benjamin, J. (1999), Recognition and destruction: An outline of inter-subjectivity (1990). In: *Relational Psychoanalysis: The Emergence of a Tradition*, ed. S. A. Mitchell & L. Aron. Hillsdale, NJ: The Analytic Press, pp. 181–210.

Bergmann, M. S. (1983), Therapeutic issues in the treatment of holocaust survivors and their children. *Amer. J. Soc. Psychiatry*, 3:21–58.

Bergmann, M. S. (1985), Reflection on the psychological and social function of remembering the Holocaust. *Psychoanal. Inq.*, 5:9–20.

Berlin, I. (1991), *The Crooked Timber of Humanity: Chapters in the History of Ideas*. New York: Knopf.

Bick, E. (1968), The experience of the skin in early object relations. *Internat. J. Psychoanal.*, 49:484–486.

Bilton, M. & Sim, K. (1992), *Four Hours in My Lai*. New York: Viking Press.

Bion, W. R. (1962), *Learning from Experience*. New York: Basic Books.

Bion, W. R. (1965), *Transformation*. London: Tavistock.

Bollas, C. (1989), The trauma of incest. *Forces of Destiny: Psychoanalysis and Human Idiom*. London: Free Association Books.

Bollas, C. (1992), *The Fascist State of Mind—Being a Character: Psychoanalysis and Self-Experience*. New York: Hill & Wang.

Bollas, C. (1995), The structure of evil. In: *Cracking Up: The Work of Unconscious Experience*. New York: Hill & Wang.

Brenneis, C. B. (1994), Memories of childhood sexual abuse. *J. Amer. Psychoanal. Assn.*, 42:1027–1055.

Brink, A. (1982), *A Chain of Voices*. New York: Penguin.

Bromberg, P. M. (1984), Getting into oneself and out of one's self: On schizoid process. *Contemp. Psychoanal.*, 11:289–303.

Bromberg, P. M. (1993), Shadow and substance: A relational perspective on clinical process. *Psychoanal. Psychol.*, 2:147–168.

Bromberg, P. M. (1994), "Speak! That I may see you." Some reflections on dissociation, reality, and psychoanalytic listening. *Contemp. Psychoanal.*, 4:517–549.

Bromberg, P. M. (1995), Psychoanalysis, dissociation, and personality organization: Reflections on Peter Goldberg's essay. *Psychoanal. Dial.*, 3:511–528.

Bromberg, P. M. (1998), *Standing in the Spaces: Essays on Clinical Process, Trauma, and Dissociation*. Hillsdale, NJ: The Analytic Press.

Brown, R. M. (1998), in Book Two: The Symposium, ed. H. J. Cargas & B. V. Fetterman. In: *The Sunflower: On the Possibilities and Limits of Forgiveness*, by S. Wiesenthal. New York: Schocken Books, pp. 121–124.

Buber, M. (1923), *I and Thou*, trans. W. Kaufman. New York: Charles Scribner's Sons, 1970.

Buber, M. (1947), *Between Man and Man*, trans. R. G. Smith. London: Routledge & Kegan Paul.

Bucci, W. (1994), The multiple code theory and the psychoanalytic process: A framework for research. *The Annual of Psychoanalysis*, 22:239–259. Hillsdale, NJ: The Analytic Press.

Camus, A. (1946), *The Stranger*. New York: Knopf.

Camus, A. (1955), *The Myth of Sisyphus*. New York: Knopf.

Camus, A. (1956), *The Fall*. New York: Knopf.

Caruth, C. (1995), Introduction. In: *Trauma: Explorations in Memory*, ed. C. Caruth. Baltimore, MD: Johns Hopkins University Press, pp. 3–13.

Chapman, A. (1968), *Black Voices*. New York: New American Library.

Chused, J. (1991), The evocative power of enactments. *J. Amer. Psychoanal. Assn.*, 39:615–639.

Clarke, B. H. (1997), Hermeneutics and the "relational" turn: Schafer, Ricoeur, Gadamer, and the nature of psychoanalytic subjectivity. *Psychoanal. Contemp. Thought*, 1:3–69.

Coltart, N. (1986), Thinking the unthinkable in psychoanalysis. In: *The British School of Psychoanalysis: The Independent Tradition*, ed. G. Kohon. New Haven, CT: Yale University Press, pp. 185–199.

Coser, L. (1969), The visibility of evil. *J. Social Issues*, 1:101–109.

Courtois, C. (1988), *Healing the Incest Wound: Adult Survivors in Therapy*. New York: Norton.

Dalai Lama (1998), in Book Two: The Symposium, ed. H. J. Cargas & B. V. Fettterman. In: *The Sunflower: On the Possibilities and Limits of Forgiveness*, by S. Wiesenthal. New York: Schocken, pp. 129–130.

Davies, J. & Frawley, M. G. (1994), *Treating the Adult Survivor of Childhood Sexual Abuse: A Psychoanalytical Perspective*. New York: Basic Books.

Dimen, M. (1998), Polyglot bodies: Thinking through the relational. In:

*Relational Perspectives on the Body*, ed. L. Aron & F. S. Anderson. Hillsdale, NJ: The Analytic Press, pp. 65–93.

Douglass, F. (1845), *Narrative of the Life of Frederick Douglass, An American Slave*. Cambridge, MA: Belknap Press of Harvard University Press, 1960.

Ehrenberg, D. (1987), Abuse and desire: A case of father–daughter incest. *Contemp. Psychoanal.*, 25:593–604.

Eigen, M. (1996), *Psychic Deadness*. Northvale, NJ: Aronson.

Eigen, M. (1998), Wilfrid, R. Bion: Infinite surfaces, explosiveness, faith. In: *Psychoanalytic Versions of the Human Condition*. New York: New York University Press, pp. 183–206.

Eliot, T. S. (1922). The wasteland. In: *T. S. Eliot, Collected Poems, 1909–1962*. New York: Harcourt, Brace & World.

Enright, R. (1991), The moral development of forgiveness. In: *Handbook of Moral Behavior and Development, Vol. 1*, ed. W. Kurtines & J. Gewirtz. Hillsdale, NJ: Lawrence Erlbaum Associates, pp. 123–152.

Epstein, L. (1977), The therapeutic function of hate in the countertransference. *Contemp. Psychoanal.*, 13:442–461.

Epstein, L. (1984), An interpersonal-object relations perspective on working with destructive aggression. *Contemp. Psychoanal.*, 20:651–662.

Fairbairn, W. R. D. (1952a), *An Object Relations Theory of the Personality*. New York: Basic Books.

Fairbairn, W. R. D. (1952b), *Psychoanalytic Studies of the Personality*. London: Routledge & Kegan Paul.

Feiner, A. H. (1995), Laughter among the peartrees: Vengeance, vindictiveness and vindication. *Contemp. Psychoanal.*, 3:381–398.

Felman, S. (1992), Education and crisis, or the vicissitudes of teaching. In *Testimony: Crises of Witnessing in Literature, Psychoanalysis, and History*, ed. S. Felman & D. Laub. New York: Routledge, 1992.

Fenichel, O. (1928), The clinical aspect of the need for punishment. *Internat. J. Psycho-Anal.*, 9:47–70.

Ferenczi, S. (1932), *The Clinical Diary of Sandor Ferenczi,* ed. J. Dupont. Cambridge, MA: Harvard University Press, 1988.

Foucault, M. (1980), *Power/Knowledge: Selected Interviews and Other Writings*, ed. C. Gordon. New York: Pantheon Books.

Fox-Genovese, E. (1988), *Within the Plantation Household: Black and White Women of the Old South*. Chapel Hill: The University of North Carolina Press.

Frankel, J. B. (1998), Ferenczi's trauma theory. *Amer. J. Psychoanal.*, 1:41–61.

Frederickson, J. (1990), Hate in the countertransference as an empathic position. *Contemp. Psychoanal.*, 26:479–497.

Fresco, N. (1984), Remembering the unknown. *Internat. Rev. Psycho-Anal*, 11:417–427.

Freud, A. (1966), *The Ego and the Mechanisms of Defense*. New York: International Universities Press.

Freud, S. (1917 [1915]), Mourning and melancholia. *Standard Edition*, 14:237–260. London: Hogarth Press, 1957.

Freud, S. (1920), Beyond the pleasure principle. *Standard Edition*, 18:7–64. London: Hogarth Press, 1955.

Freud, S. (1921), Group psychology and the analysis of the ego. *Standard Edition*, 18:69–143. London: Hogarth Press, 1955.

Freud, S. (1923), The ego and the id. *Standard Edition*, 19:3–68. London: Hogarth Press, 1961.

Freud, S. (1927), The future of an illusion. *Standard Edition*, 21:3–58. London: Hogarth Press, 1961.

Freud, S. (1930), Civilization and its discontents. *Standard Edition*, 21:64–145. London: Hogarth Press, 1961.

Freud, S. (1937), Analysis terminable and interminable. *Standard Edition*, 23:209–253. London: Hogarth Press, 1964.

Fromm, E. (1964), *The Heart of Man: Its Genius for Good and Evil*. New York: Harper & Row.

Fromm-Reichmann, F. (1959, rpt. 1990), Loneliness. *Contemp. Psychoanal.*, 2:305–330.

Gabbard, G. O. (1997), A reconstruction of objectivity in the analyst. *Internat. J. Psycho-Anal.*, 78:15–26.

Galdston, R. (1987), The longest pleasure: A psychoanalytic study of hatred. *Internat. J. Psycho-Anal.*, 68:371–378.

Gampel, Y. (1982), A daughter of silence. In: *Generations of the Holocaust*, ed. M. S. Bergmann & M. E. Jucovy. New York: Columbia University Press, pp. 120–137.

Gartner, R. (1999), *Betrayed as Boys*. New York: Guilford Press.

Gebhardt, B. (1970), *Handbuch der Deutschen Geschichte, Vol. 4*. Stuttgart: Klettcotta.

Geha, R. (1993), Transferred fictions. *Psychoanal. Dial.*, 3:209–245.

Genovese, E. D. (1972), *Roll, Jordan, Roll: The World the Slaves Made*. New York: Vintage Books.

Ghent, E. (1992), Paradox and process. *Psychoanal. Dial.*, 2:135–160.

Gill, M. M. (1982), *The Analysis of Transference, Vol. 1*. New York: International Universities Press.

Gill, M. M. (1995), Classical and relational psychoanalysis. *Psychoanal. Psychol.*, 12:89–108.

Gilligan, J. (1992), *Violence*. New York: G. P. Putnam's Sons.

Goldberg, C. (1996), *Speaking with the Devil: A Dialogue with Evil*. New York: Viking.

Goldberg, P. (1987), The role of distractions in the maintenance of dissociative mental states. *Internat. J. Psycho-Anal.*, 68:511–524.

Goldhagen, D. J. (1996), *Hitler's Willing Executioners*. New York: Knopf.

Goldner, V. (1998), The treatment of violence and victimization in intimate relationships. *Family Process*, 1:263–286.

Grand, S. (1995), Incest and the intersubjective politics of knowing history. In: *Sexual Abuse Recalled: Treating Trauma in the Era of the Recovered Memory Debate*, ed. J. Alpert. Northvale, NJ: Aronson, pp. 235–253.

Grand, S. (1997a), On the gendering of traumatic dissociation: A case of mother-son incest. *Gender & Psychoanal.*, 1:55–79.

Grand, S. (1997b), The paradox of innocence: Dissociative "adhesive" states in perpetrators of incest. *Psychoanal. Dial.*, 4:465–491.

Grand, S. & Alpert, J. (1993), The core trauma of incest: An object relations view. *Professional Psychol. Res. Prac.*, 24:330–334.

Greenberg, J. R. (1999), Theoretical models and the analyst's neutrality. In: *Relational Psychoanalysis: The Emergence of a Tradition*, ed. S. A. Mitchell & L. Aron. Hillsdale, NJ: The Analytic Press, pp. 133–152.

Greenberg, J. R. & Mitchell, S. A. (1983), *Object Relations in Psychoanalytic Theory*. Cambridge, MA: Harvard University Press.

Groth, A. N. (1982), The incest offender. In: *The Handbook of Clinical Intervention in Child Sexual Abuse*, ed. S. M. Sgroi. Lexington, MA: Heath.

Grotstein, J. S. (1979), Demonical possession, splitting and the torment of joy. *Contemp. Psychoanal.*, 3:407–445.

Grotstein, J. S. (1981), *Splitting and Projective Identification*. Northvale, NJ: Aronson.

Grotstein, J. S. (1990), Nothingness, meaninglessness, chaos and "the Black Hole" II. *Contemp. Psychoanal.*, 3:377–408.

Guntrip, H. (1969), *Schizoid Phenomena, Object Relations and the Self*. New York: International Universities Press.

Guntrip, H. (1971), *Psychoanalytic Theory, Therapy and the Self*. New York: Basic Books.

Hammer, R. (1971), *The Court Martial of Lieutenant Calley*. New York: Coward, McCann, & Geoghegan.

Harris, A. (1994), Gender practices and speech practices: Towards a model of dialogical and relational selves. Presented at annual meeting of the American Psychological Association, Division 39, Washington, DC.

Harris, A. (1996), Animated conversation: Embodying and engendering. *Gender & Psychoanal*, 1:361–384.

Harris, A. (1997). Deconstructing the false memory syndrome. In: *Memories of Sexual Betrayal*, ed. R. Gartner. Northvale, NJ: Aronson.

Harris, A. (1998), Psychic envelopes and sonorous baths: Sitting the body in relational theory and clinical practice. In: *Relational Perspectives on the Body*, ed. L. Aron & F. S. Anderson. Hillsdale, NJ: The Analytic Press, pp. 39–64.

Hayashino, D. S., Wurtele, S. K. & Klebe, K. J. (1995), Child molesters: An examination of cognitive factors. *J. Interpersonal Violence*, 10:106–116.

Hegemon, E. (1995), Transferential issues in the psychoanalytic treatment of incest survivors. In: *Sexual Abuse Recalled*, ed. J. Alpert. Northvale, NJ: Aronson.

Heidegger, M. (1962), *Being and Time*. New York: Harper & Row.

Herman, J. L. (1992), *Trauma and Recovery*. New York: Basic Books.

Herman, J. L. & Harvey, M. R. (1993). The false memory debate: Social science or social backlash? *Harvard Mental Health Newsletter* 9:4–6.

Hirsch, I. (1993), Countertransference enactments and some issues related to external factors in the analyst's life. *Psychoanal. Dial.*, 3:343–366.

Hoffman, I. Z. (1992), Reply to Orange. *Psychoanal. Dial.*, 2:567–570.

Hopper, E. (1995), The incohesion basic assumption. Paper presented at a panel on the narcissistic group leader at the annual scientific meeting of the American Group Psychotherapy Association, Atlanta, GA, February.

Horney, K. (1948), The value of vindictiveness. *Amer. J. Psychoanal.*, 8:3–12.

Hoss, R. (1946), Autobiography of Rudolf Hoss. In: *KL Auschwitz Seen by the SS*, ed. J. Bezwinska & D. Czech. New York: Fertig, 1994.

Howell, E. F. (1996), Dissociation in masochism and psychopathic sadism. *Contemp. Psychoanal.*, 3:427–455.

Jacobs, T. J. (1986), On countertransference enactments. *J. Amer. Psychoanal. Assn.*, 34:289–307.

Kafka, H. (1995), Incestuous sexual abuse, memory, and the organization of the self. In: *Sexual Abuse Recalled*, ed. J. Alpert. Northvale, NJ: Aronson, pp. 135–155.

Kestenberg, J. (1982), Survivor-parents and their children. In: *Generations of the Holocaust*, ed. M. S. Bergmann & M. E. Jucovy. New York: Columbia University Press, pp. 83–101.

Kierkegaard, S. (1937), *The Concept of Dread*. Princeton, NJ: Princeton University Press.

King, M. L., Jr. (1963), *I Have a Dream*, ed. J. M. Washington. San Francisco: Harper, 1986.

Klein, M. (1935), A contribution to the psychogenesis of manic-depressive states. In: *Contributions to Psychoanalysis, 1921–1945*. London: Hogarth Press, pp. 282–311.

Klein, M. (1940), Mourning and its relation to manic-depressive states. *Internat. J. Psycho-Anal.*, 21:125–153.

Klein, M. (1946), Notes on some schizoid mechanisms. In: *Developments in Psychoanalysis*, ed. M. Klein, P. Heimann, S. Isaacs & J. Riviere. London: Hogarth Press, 1952, pp. 292–320.

Klein, M. (1948), On the theory of anxiety and guilt. In: *Envy and Gratitude and Other Works, 1946–1963*. New York: Delacorte, 1975, pp. 25–42.

Klein, M. (1955), On identification. In: *Envy and Gratitude and Other Works, 1946–1963*. New York: Delacorte, 1975, pp. 176–234.

Klein, M. (1983), On the theory of anxiety and guilt. In: *Developments in Psychoanalysis*, ed. M. Klein, P. Heimann, S. Isaacs & J. Riviere. New York: De Capo Press, pp. 271–292.

Klein, M. & Riviere, J. (1964), *Love, Hate and Reparation*. New York: W. W. Norton.

Kramer, S. (1983), Object-coercive doubting: A pathological defensive response to maternal incest. *J. Amer. Psychoanal. Assn.*, 31:325–351.

Kreegman, S. (1987), Trauma in the family: Perspectives on the intergenerational transmission of violence. In: *Psychological Trauma*, ed. B. A. Van der Kolk. Washington, DC: American Psychiatric Press, pp. 127–152.

Kristeva, J. (1980), Powers of horror. In *The Portable Kristeva*, ed. K. Oliver. New York: Columbia University Press, 1997, pp. 229–264.

Krystal, H. (1976), Trauma and affect. *The Psychoanalytic Study of the Child*, 33:81–116. New York: International Universities Press.

Krystal, H. (1988), *Integration and Self-Healing: Affect, Trauma, Alexithymia*. Hillsdale, NJ: The Analytic Press.

Laing, R. D. (1960), *The Divided Self*. New York: Penguin Books.

Langer, L. (1991), *Holocaust Testimonies: The Ruins of Memory*. New Haven, CT: Yale University Press.

Langer, L. (1995), *Admitting the Holocaust*. New York: Oxford University Press.

Langer, L. (1998), in Book Two: The Symposium, ed. H. J. Cargas & B. V. Fetterman. In *The Sunflower: On the Possibilities and Limits of Forgiveness*, by S. Wiesenthal. New York: Schocken, pp. 186–190.

Lanzmann, C. (1995). The obscenity of understanding: An evening with Claude Lanzmann. In: *Trauma: Explorations in Memory*, ed. C. Caruth. Baltimore: Johns Hopkins University Press.

Laub, D. (1992), Bearing witness, or the vicissitudes of listening. In: *Testimony: Crises of Witnessing in Literature, Psychoanalysis, and History*, ed. S. Felman & D. Laub. New York: Routledge.

Laub, D. & Auerhahn, N. C. (1989), Failed empathy: A central theme in the survivor's Holocaust experience. *Psychoanal. Psychol.*, 6:377–400.

Laub, D. & Auerhahn, N. C. (1993), Knowing and not-knowing massive psychic trauma: Forms of traumatic memory. *Internat. J. Psycho-Anal.*, 74:287–302.

Laub, D. & Podell, D. (1995), Art and trauma. *Internat. J. Psycho-Anal.*, 76:991–1005.

Liegner, E. J. (1980), The hate that cures: The psychological reversibility of schizophrenia. *Mod. Psychoanal.*, 5:5–95.

Lifton, R. J. (1961), *Thought Control and the Psychology of Totalism*. New York: W. W. Norton.

Lifton, R. J. (1986), *The Nazi Doctors*. New York: Basic Books.

Lifton, R. J. (1996), Dreaming well: On death and history. In: *Trauma and Dreams*, ed. D. Barrett. London: Harvard University Press, pp. 125–140.

Lifton, R. J. & Markhusen, E. (1990), *The Genocidal Mentality*. New York: Basic Books.

Lindsay, D. S. & Read, J. D. (1994), Psychotherapy and memories of childhood sexual abuse: A cognitive perspective. *Appl. Cognitive Psychol.*, 8:281–339.

Lionells, M. (1992), Things aren't what they used to be, but then, they never were. *Contemp. Psychoanal.*, 28:309–326.

Little, M. I. (1985), *Psychotic Anxieties and Containment*. Northvale, NJ: Aronson.

Loewenstein, R. M. (1956), Some remarks on the role of speech in psychoanalytic technique. *Internat. J. Psycho-Anal.*, 37:460–468.

Loftus, E. (1991). *Witness for the Defense*. New York: St. Martin's.

Lynn, S. J. & Nash, M. R. (1994), Truth in memory: Ramifications for psychotherapy and hypnotherapy. *Amer. J. Clin. Hypnosis*, 36, No. 3.

Maas, P. (1996), *Love Thy Neighbor: A Story of War*. New York: Vintage Books.

MacLaughlin, J. (1991), Clinical and theoretical aspects of enactment. *J. Amer. Psychoanal. Assn.*, 39:595–614.

May, R. (1981), *Freedom and Destiny*. New York: W. W. Norton.

McDougall, J. (1989), *Theaters of the Body: A Psychoanalytic Approach to Psychosomatic Illness*. New York: W. W. Norton.

McGinn, C. (1997), *Ethics, Evil and Fiction*. Oxford: Clarendon Press.

Meltzer, D. (1975), Adhesive identification. *Contemp. Psychoanal.*, 11:289–303.

Michaels, A. (1997), *Fugitive Pieces*. New York: Knopf.

Mitchell, S. (1993a), Aggression and the endangered self. *Psychoanal. Quart.*, 62:351–382.

Mitchell, S. (1993b), *Hope and Dread in Psychoanalysis*. New York: Basic Books.

Mitchell, S. (1995), Interaction in the Kleinian and interpersonal traditions. *Contemp. Psychoanal.*, 31:65–91.

Mitrani, J. (1994a), On adhesive pseudo–object relations, part I. *Contemp. Psychoanal.*, 30:348–367.

Mitrani, J. (1994b), On adhesive pseudo–object relations, part II. *Contemp. Psychoanal.*, 31:140–165.

Nachmani, G. (1995), Trauma and ignorance. *Contemp. Psychoanal.*, 3:423–451.

Nachmani, G. (1997), Discussion: Reconstructing the methods of victimization. In: *Memories of Sexual Betrayal*, ed. R. Gartner. Northvale, NJ: Aronson, pp. 189–209.

O'Brian, T. (1990), *The Things They Carried*. New York: Penguin Books.

Ogden, T. (1989), *The Primitive Edge of Experience*. Northvale, NJ: Aronson.

Ogden, T. (1990), *The Matrix of the Mind*. Northvale, NJ: Aronson.

Ogden, T. (1994), *Subjects of Analysis*. Northvale, NJ: Aronson.

Ogden, T. (1997), *Reverie and Imagination: Sensing Something Human*. Northvale, NJ: Aronson.

Orwell, G. (1949), *1984*. New York: Harcourt Brace Jovanovich.

O'Shaughnessy, E. (1990), Can a liar be psychoanalysed? *Internat. J. Psycho-Anal.*, 71:187–195.

Owens, W. (1953), *A Black Mutiny*. New York: Plume Books.

Ozick, C. (1998), in Book Two: The Symposium, ed. H. J. Cargas & B. V. Fetterman. In: *The Sunflower: On the Possibilities and Limits of Forgiveness*, by S. Wiesenthal. New York: Schocken, pp. 213–220.

Pao, P. N. (1965), The role of hatred in the ego. *Psychoanal. Quart.*, 34:257–264.

Pavlikowski, J. J. (1998), in Book Two: The Symposium, ed. H. J. Cargas & B. V. Fetterman. In: *The Sunflower: On the Possibilities and Limits of Forgiveness*, by S. Wiesenthal. New York: Schocken.

Peck, M. (1983), *People of the Lie: The Hope for Healing Human Evil.* New York: Simon & Schuster.

Pizer, S. A. (1999), The negotiation of paradox in the analytic process. In: *Relational Psychoanalysis: The Emergence of a Tradition*, ed. S. A. Mitchell & L. Aron. Hillsdale, NJ: The Analytic Press, pp. 337–364.

Price, M. (1992). Incest: Transference and countertransference implications. Paper presented at the Americal Academy of Psychoanalysis, Dec.

Price, M. (1995), Knowing and not knowing: paradox in the construction of historical narratives. In: *Delayed Memories of Childhood Sexual Abuse: Treating Trauma in the Era of the Recovered Memory Debate*, ed. J. Alpert. Northvale, NJ: Aronson, pp. 289–309.

Putnam, F. W. (1990), Disturbances of "self" in victims of incest and child abuse. In: *Incest Related Syndromes of Adult Psychopathology*, ed. R. P. Kluft. Washington, DC: American Psychiatric Press, pp. 113–131.

Pye, E. (1996), Memory and imagination: Placing imagination in the therapy of individuals with incest memories. In: *Sexual Abuse Recalled*, ed. J. L. Alpert. Northvale, NJ: Aronson, pp. 155–185.

Rank, O. (1936), *Will Therapy and Truth and Reality.* New York: Knopf.

Rappaport, D. (1998), Destruction and gratitude: Some thoughts on "the use of an object." *Contemp. Psychoanal.*, 34:369–378.

Reis, B. (1993), Toward a psychoanalytic understanding of multiple personality disorder. *Bull. Menn. Clin.*, 57:309–318.

Reis, B. (1995), The incest perpetrator's use of dissociative projective identification: The space of malignant transformation. Unpublished manuscript.

Renik, O. (1993), Countertransference enactment and the psychoanalytic process. In: *Psychic Structure and Psychic Change*, ed. M. Horowitz, O. Kernberg & E. Weinshel. Madison, CT: International Universities Press, pp. 135–158.

Riviere, J. (1964), *Love, Hate, and Reparation.* New York: W. W. Norton.

Robins, R. S. & Post, J. M. (1997), *The Psychopolitics of Hatred.* New Haven, CT: Yale University Press.

Safer, J. (1999), *Forgiving and Not Forgiving.* New York: Avon.

Sampson, H. (1992), The role of "real" experience in psychopathology and treatment. *Psychoanal. Dial.*, 2:509–529.

Sartre, J. P. (1956), *Being and Nothingness*, trans. H. E. Barnes. New York: Philosophical Library.

Sartre, J. P. (1981), *Existential Psychoanalysis*. Washington, DC: Regnery.

Sass, L. A. (1993). Psychoanalysis as "conversations" and as "fictions": A commentary on Charles Spezzano's "A relational model of inquiry and truth" and Richard Geha's "Transferred fictions." *Psychoanal. Dial.*, 3:245–255.

Scarry, E. (1985), *The Body in Pain*. New York: Oxford University Press.

Schachtel, E. (1959), *Metamorphosis: On the Development of Affect, Perception, Attention and Memory*. New York: Basic Books.

Schafer, R. (1983), *The Analytic Attitude*. New York: Basic Books.

Schlesinger-Silver, A. L. (1990), Resuming the work with a life-threatening illness, and further reflections. In: *Illness in the Analyst*, ed, H. J. Schwartz & A. L. Schlesinger-Silver. New York: International Universities Press, pp. 151–177.

Schwartz, H. J. (1990), Illness in the doctor: Implications for the psychoanalytic process. In: *Illness in the Analyst*, ed. H. J. Schwartz & A. L. Schlesinger-Silver. New York: International Universities Press, pp. 115–151.

Searles, H. F. (1956), The psychodynamics of vengefulness. *Psychiatry*, 19:31–39.

Searles, H. F. (1959), The effort to drive the other person crazy: An element in the aetiology and psychotherapy of schizophrenia. In: *Collected Papers on Schizophrenia and Related Subjects*. New York: International Universities Press, 1965, pp. 254–283.

Searles, H. F. (1960), *The Nonhuman Environment*. Madison, CT: International Universities Press.

Segal, H. (1957), Notes on symbol formation. *Internat. J. Psycho-Anal.*, 38:391–397.

Segal, H. (1964), *Introduction to the Work of Melanie Klein*. New York: Basic Books.

Shakespeare, W. (n.d.), *Hamlet, Prince of Denmark*. New York: Penguin Books, 1957.

Shakespeare, W. (n.d.), *Macbeth*. New York: Routledge, 1951.

Shapiro, S. (1997), Discussion: Makes me want to shout. In: *Memories of Sexual Betrayal*, ed. R. Gartner. Northvale, NJ: Aronson, pp. 95–113.

Shatan, C. (1977), Bogus manhood, bogus honor: Surrender and transformation in the U.S. Marine Corps. *Psychoanal. Rev.*, 4:585–610.

Shatan, C. (1982), The tattered ego of survivors. *Psychiatric Annals,* 11:1031–1038.

Shatan, C. (1986), Afterword: Who can take away the wound. In: *The Vietnam Veteran Redefined: Fact and Fiction,* ed. G. Boulanger & C. Kadushin. Hillsdale, NJ: Lawrence Erlbaum Associates.

Shelley, M. (1818), *Frankenstein.* New York: Dell, 1965.

Shengold, L. (1989), *Soul Murder: The Effects of Childhood Abuse and Deprivation.* New Haven, CT: Yale University Press.

Simenauer, E. (1982), The return of the persecutor. In: *Generations of the Holocaust,* ed. M. S. Bergmann & M. E. Jucovy. New York: Columbia University Press, pp. 167–176.

Slavin, J. H. (1997), Memory, dissociation, and agony in sexual abuse. In: *Memories of Sexual Betrayal,* ed. R. Gartner. Northvale, NJ: Aronson, pp. 221–237.

Slochower, J. (1996), *Holding and Psychoanalysis.* Northvale, NJ: The Analytic Press.

Socarides, C. W. (1966), On vengeance: The desire to "get even." *J. Amer. Psychoanal. Assn.,* 14:356–375.

Soyinka, W. (1999), *The Burden of Memory, The Muse of Forgiveness.* New York: Oxford University Press.

Speer, A. (1998), in Book Two: The Symposium, ed. H. J. Cargas & B. V. Fetterman. In: *The Sunflower: On the Possibilities and Limits of Forgiveness,* by S. Wiesenthal. New York: Schocken, pp. 266–268.

Spence, D. (1982), *Narrative Truth and Historical Truth.* New York: Norton.

Spence, D. (1993). The hermeneutic turn: Soft science or loyal opposition? *Psychoanal. Dial.,* 3:1–11.

Spezzano, C. (1993), A relational model of inquiry and truth: The place of psychoanalysis in human conversation. *Psychoanal. Dial.,* 3:177–209.

Staub, E. (1989), *The Roots of Evil: The Origins of Genocide and Other Group Violence.* New York: Cambridge University Press.

Stern, D. B. (1997), *Unformulated Experience: From Dissociation to Imagination in Psychoanalysis.* Hillsdale, NJ: The Analytic Press.

Stern, M. (1995), *Jung on Evil.* Princeton, NJ: Princeton University Press.

Stolorow, R. D. & Lachmann, F. M. (1980), *Psychoanalysis of Developmental Arrests.* New York: International Universities Press.

Sullivan, H. S. (1953), *The Interpersonal Theory of Psychiatry.* New York: Norton.

Thomas, D. (1952), And death shall have no dominion. In: *Collected Poems.* New York: New Directions Books.

Todorov, T. (1996), *Facing the Extreme: Moral Life in the Concentration Camp.* New York: Metropolitan Books.

Troutt, D. (1998), *The Monkey Suit.* New York: The New Press.

Tutu, D. (1998), in Book Two: The Symposium, ed. H. J. Cargas & B. V. Fetterman. In: *The Sunflower: On the Possibilities and Limits of Forgiveness*, by S. Wiesenthal. New York: Schocken, pp. 266–268.

Ulman, R. B. & Brothers, D. (1988), *The Shattered Self: A Psychoanalytic Study of Trauma.* Hillsdale, NJ: The Analytic Press.

Unsworth, B. (1992), *Sacred Hunger.* New York: Norton.

Van der Kolk, B. A. (1996), The body keeps the score: Approaches to the psychobiology of posttraumatic stress disorder. In: *Traumatic Stress*, ed. B. A. Van der Kolk, A. C. MacFarlane & L. Weisaeth. New York: Guilford, pp. 214–241.

Van Zyl, S. (1999), Interview with Gillian Straker on the truth and reconciliation commission in South Africa. *Psychoanal. Dial.*, 9:245–272.

Waite, R. G. L. (1952), *Vanguard of Nazism: The Free Corps Movement in Postwar Germany, 1918–1923.* Cambridge, MA: Harvard University Press.

Waites, E. A. (1993), *Trauma and Survival: Post Traumatic and Dissociative Disorders in Women.* New York: W. W. Norton.

Walsh, N. (1996), Life and death. In: *Trauma and Self*, ed. C. Strozier & M. Flynn. Lanham, MD: Rowman & Littlefield.

Williams, A. H. (1998), Psychotic development in a sexually abused borderline patient. *Psychoanal. Dial.*, 8:513–518.

Williams, P. (1998), Psychotic developments in a sexually abused borderline patient. *Psychoanal. Dial.*, 4:459–493.

Winnicott, D. W. (1947), Hate in the countertransference. In: *Through Paediatrics to Psychoanalysis.* London: Hogarth Press, 1958, pp. 194–204.

Winnicott, D. W. (1954), The depressive position in normal emotional development. In: *Through Paediatrics to Psychoanalysis.* London: Hogarth Press, 1958, pp. 262–278.

Winnicott, D. W. (1958). Psychoanalysis and the sense of guilt. In: *The Maturational Processes and the Facilitating Environment.* New York: International Universities Press, pp. 15–29.

Winnicott, D. W. (1960), Ego distortion in terms of true and false self. In: *The Maturational Processes and the Facilitating Environment.* New York: International Universities Press, 1965, pp. 140–152.

Winnicott, D. W. (1963), The development of the capacity for concern. In: *The Maturational Processes and the Facilitating Environment.* New

York: International Universities Press, 1965, pp. 73–82.

Wolfe, T. (1957), *The Face of a Nation*. New York: Charles Scribner's Sons.

Yalom, I. D. (1980), *Existential Psychotherapy*. New York: Basic Books.

Yeats, W. B. (1921), The second coming. In: *The Collected Poems of W. B. Yeats*. New York: Macmillan, 1933.

# INDEX